TABLE OF CONTENTS:

How to use this Book ix

Supplies List 1

NingXia Red Shots... 2

My YL Now What? Bundles... 4

Now What? Wellness 101 Script... 8

Cardiovascular / Circulatory Systems Script............................. 20

Digestive / Excretory Systems Script 30

Endocannabinoid System Script 40

Endocrine / Reproductive Systems Script 50

Integumentary / Exocrine System Script 60

Immune / Lymphatic / Respiratory Systems Script 68

Musculoskeletal System Script 78

Nervous System Script 86

Renal / Urinary System Script.. 96

FOREWORD

The book Now What? explored some very practical ways for the average person to support, maintain, and promote a vibrant, healthy immune system in the short time-frame of only four months. Members using the Now What? book though, needed a simple way to share and instruct on the principles found within. This simple book, Now What? Scripts, fills that void. Now What? Scripts takes us step by step through sharing product opportunity with each system of the body, providing an easy way to share Young Living products using scripts based off of the Now What? book. Today we live in a world where, through governmental restrictions, we find ourselves at a loss on what to say for fear of the protecting ourselves and the Young Living brand. This book removes that fear and replaces it with an easy, duplicable way to share.

I often hear people say, "I just need a system to follow." The Now What? book series is for anyone looking to take charge of his or her life. Wellness seeks more than the absence of illness; it searches for new levels of excellence. Winning strategies that work are incredibly simple. The more complicated, harder something is, the more ego or untruth that is present. The scripts are simple, easy, and fun. Ultimately, this book is about empowering you to become more confident, more independent, and wiser thinkers when sharing Young Living. Mastering how to share Young Living and how to influence and persuade others through connecting them with their own bodies and with an integral company, Young Living, will generate top-producing business results. Susan and Bobbi are inspirational leaders in creating a high standard for mentoring, coaching, and supporting all who choose to step up in their own wellness goals.

~Marcella Vonn Harting, PhD

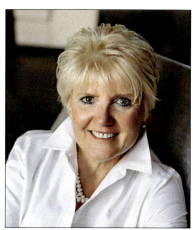

How to use the
NOW WHAT? SCRIPTS BOOK

Thank you for investing in your *Now What? Scripts* book. We are happy that you have made this commitment to your health and the health of the people who are important to you.

You now hold in your hands an extraordinary resource for teaching Young Living wellness classes, building your business, and navigating your own health goals. Each script goes over the essential oil-infused products, specific to each body system, in an easy to teach class format. This will aid you and your customers in making informed decisions on how to personalize your 4-Month Wellness Plans.

We wrote this book to be the perfect class companion to help you fully utilize your Now What? book. It is meant to empower YOU with scientifically validated information that will assist you in personalizing and designing a plan to meet your health goals or the health goals of attendees in your classes. You can now easily teach your friends and your team about the products listed for each of the body systems, offering you a roadmap to what, why, and when to get them.

The first script is for your Now What? Wellness 101 class. Each subsequent script correlates with each of the body systems in your Now What? book. Regardless of the class you are teaching, you will notice NingXia Red is the foundation of each plan and script. We have also included Vitality Dietary Oils and Targeted Supplements for each body system. In addition, there is a bonus section on products "You May Also Like". Many of these products also correlate with products under the You May Also Like section on each product page found on the Young Living shopping platform. Move this sentence after "Regardless of the class you are teaching, you will notice NingXia Red is the foundation of each plan and script. So, whether you are teaching a 101 wellness class, a product education class for your team, or simply sharing with a friend, you have exactly what you need at your fingertips.

We know you've been talking to your family and friends about how the Young Living products have helped you. And, we recognize that sometimes it is hard to help them navigate this process. With the Now What? and the Now What? Scripts books, we have taken the guesswork out and given you a resource to easily walk them through the process of personalizing their Subscribe to Save Order and 4-Month Wellness Plan.

So, with that in mind, let's talk about the process of how this works in a class setting.

First, make a list of everyone you know and everyone you meet along the way that can benefit from the Young Living products. And let's be clear, EVERYONE you know and meet can benefit from these products. Start making calls to invite everyone from this list to a Now What? class.

To keep it personal, the perfect sized Now What? class is 6-10 attendees. Remember to pre-qualify your guests. If they are not interested or with another company, they are not qualified guests. Confirming their attendance should be done 72 and 24 hours prior to the event.

At your Now What? class, there is a specific etiquette to follow: dress professionally, show your passion, be enthusiastic, present with confidence, build relationships, show your gratitude, and SMILE. Show up 125% and know you are providing a much needed service for your friends, so listen carefully to their needs, meet them where they are, and close with confidence.

Food at a class is a distraction; instead we recommend offering a NingXia Red shot appropriate to the body system from which you are teaching (see page 2). If you feel you need to serve something additional during the class, you can serve water infused with a Vitality Oil or a snack from the Young Living catalogue.

Have a sign in sheet available, and as your guests arrive, have them sign in. Be sure to collect their names, phone numbers, and emails. You will use this information to follow up with everyone. (This is the hostess's responsibility.)

The scripts are designed to take, at most, 30 minutes to present. At the beginning of each class, you will provide each guest with their own Now What? book. (This, also is the hostess's responsibility. Be sure to fill in the appropriate Sponsor Member#, Member Phone# and the My Member#, My Pin# and My Password section on the back of each book). If this is a basic wellness class, you will give the book to each guest and let them know what system of the body their health goal is related to. If it is a system specific class, instruct them to open their Now What? book to the corresponding page.

Now... READ THE SCRIPT, have FUN and bring your personality. Once you have finished reading the script, simply direct them to the appropriate "4 Month Wellness Plan" section to personalize their plans. Have them pull out their smartphones or tablets and help them set up their order. You can also set up bundles in advance on your My YL Website (see page 4). Send the attendees the link to this bundle to easily choose the products they want to order and set up on Subscribe to Save.

After the class, follow up with each guest. Your mission is to help them with their wellness goals. You do this by enrolling them and helping them get on Subscribe to Save with a 4-Month Wellness Plan.

This book can also be used as a personal guide for your own wellness goals. Pick a system of the body YOU want to support, and use Now What? and the Now What? Script book to educate and empower yourself in creating your own wellness plan.

We are looking forward to hearing your success stories. Please share them on our Facebook Page at Now What? or on Instagram @NowWhatYL.

 Now What?
 NowWhatYL

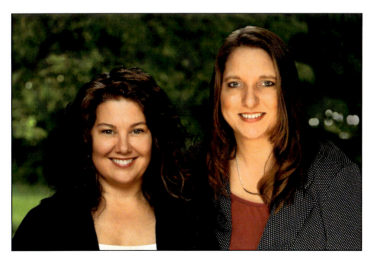

Bobbi Decker and Susan Richardson

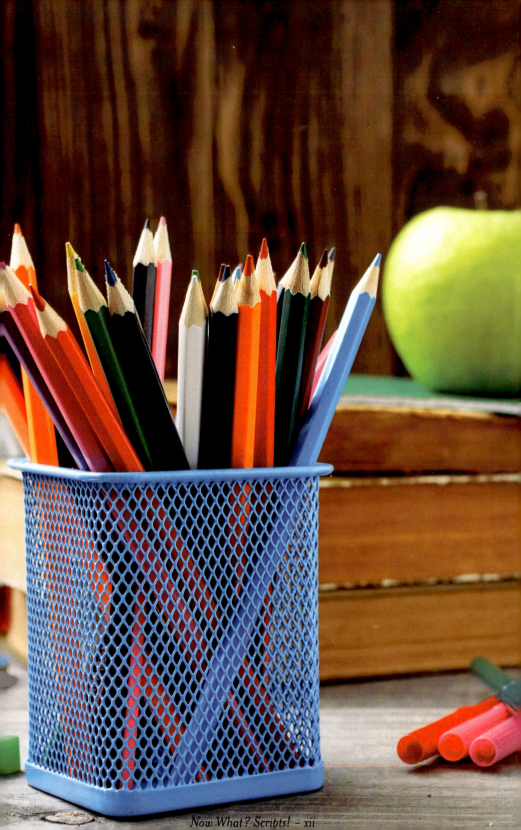

SUPPLIES LIST
for your Introductory Class, Meeting or Workshop

- Now What? books (one for each guest)
- Essential Oils listed in the Now What? section you are teaching on
- NingXia Red and cups or shot glasses
- Thieves Products of choice
- Everyday Oils Kit
- V-6
- 32 ounce spray bottle
- Sign-in sheet
- Sticky notes
- Pens
- Pad of paper
- 4 or more product guides (labeled 'demo copy')
- Laptop or tablet
- List of your next 3 classes and your calendar

NOW WHAT?

NINGXIA RED
SYSTEM SUPPORTING SHOTS

Cardio/Circulatory Systems (spicy)

- 1 oz NingXia Red®
- 1 drop Cinnamon Bark Vitality™
- 2 drops Orange Vitality™

Digestive System

- 1 oz NingXia Red
- 1 drop Fennel Vitality™
- 1 drop Tangerine Vitality™

Endocannabinoid System

- 1 oz Ningxia Red
- 1 drop Black Pepper Vitality
- 1 drop Orange Vitality

Integumentary System

- 1 oz NingXia Red
- 1 drop Fennel Vitality
- 1 drop Tangerine Vitality

Respiratory/Immune Systems (spicy)

- 1 oz NingXia Red
- 1 drop Thieves Vitality™
- 2 drops Orange Vitality™

Endocrine/Reproductive Systems

- 1 oz NingXia Red
- 1 drop Lemon Vitality™
- 1 drop Frankincense Vitality™

Musculoskeletal System

- 1 oz NingXia Red
- 1 drop Lemongrass Vitality™
- 1 drop Copaiba Vitality™

Nervous System

- 1 oz NingXia Red
- 1 drop Lavender Vitality™
- 1 drop Frankincense Vitality

Urinary System

- 1 oz NingXia Red
- 1 drop Lemon Vitality
- 1 drop Grapefruit Vitality™
- 3 droppers K& B

MY YL NOW WHAT? BUNDLES

Your new Brand Partners will get a free 3 month subscription to the MY YL Website in their Business Essentials Kit. We encourage you and your Brand Partners to use the "Manage Enroll With Me" option to customize multiple enrollment links with Now What? bundles based on the classes you are teaching from this book. You can text these links to individuals, class attendees, or use them on social media.

Cardiovascular System Bundle
- NingXia Red
- MindWise
- OmegaGize3
- Cinnamon Bark Vitality
- Aroma Life
- Super B
- CardioGize

Digestive System Bundle
- NingXia Red
- 5 Day Nutritive Cleanse
- Sulfurzyme Powder
- Life 9
- AlkaLime
- Balance Complete
- Allerzyme

Endocannabinoid System Bundle
- NingXia Red
- Natures Ultra Citrus CBD
- Natures Ultra Cool Mint CBD
- Natures Ultra Cinnamon CBD
- Natures Ultra Calm CBD Roll-on
- Natures Ultra CBD Muscle Rub
- Mineral Essence
- Life 9
- OmegaGize3
- Super D

Endocrine System (Women) Bundle
- NingXia Red
- FemiGen
- PD 80/20
- Super B
- Cortistop
- Dragon Time Bath and Shower Gel
- Pure Protein Plus
- Clary Sage
- EndoFlex
- Progessence Plus

Endocrine System (Men) Bundle
- NingXia Red
- Master Formula
- Prostate Health
- Mister
- Charcoal Bar Soap
- Shutran
- PowerGize
- Super B
- Idaho Blue Spruce

Integumentary Bundle
- NingXia Red
- Super B
- Life 9
- Sulfurzyme Powder
- Lavender Shampoo
- Orange Blossom Facial Wash
- Orange Blossom Facial Moisturizer
- Essentialzyme
- Lavender Bath & Body Gel
- Mirah Shave Oil

MY YL NOW WHAT? BUNDLES

Immune System Bundle
- NingXia Red
- Life 9
- Inner Defense
- Thieves Household Cleaner
- Thieves Foaming Hand Wash
- Thieves Hand Sanitizer
- Thieves Dish Soap
- Thieves Vitality
- Super C
- MultiGreens

Musculoskeletal Bundle
- NingXia Red
- AgilEase
- PowerGize
- OmegaGize3
- MindWise
- OTC Cool Azul Pain Cream
- AminoWise
- Nature's Ultra CBD Joint and Muscle Rub
- Lemongrass Vitality
- Copaiba Vitality

Nervous Bundle
- NingXia Red
- MindWise
- NingXia Nitro
- OmegaGize3
- Brain Power
- Mineral Essence
- AminoWise
- Thieves Household Cleaner
- Lavender Shampoo
- Sacred Frankincense

Renal/Urinary System Bundle
- NingXia Red
- K & B
- Balance Complete
- ImmuPro
- Inner Defense
- Life 9
- Lemon Vitality
- Grapefruit Vitality
- Super B
- Master Formula

Reproductive System Bundle
- NingXia Red
- Master Formula
- Shutran
- FemiGen
- Prostate Health
- PD 80/20
- Progessence Plus
- EndoGize
- Sensation Massage Oil
- Jasmine

Respiratory System Bundle
- NingXia Red
- MultiGreens
- Inner Defense
- Life 9
- Thieves Household Cleaning
- Thieves Hand Sanitizer
- Super C
- RC
- Lemon Vitality
- Eucalyptus Radiata

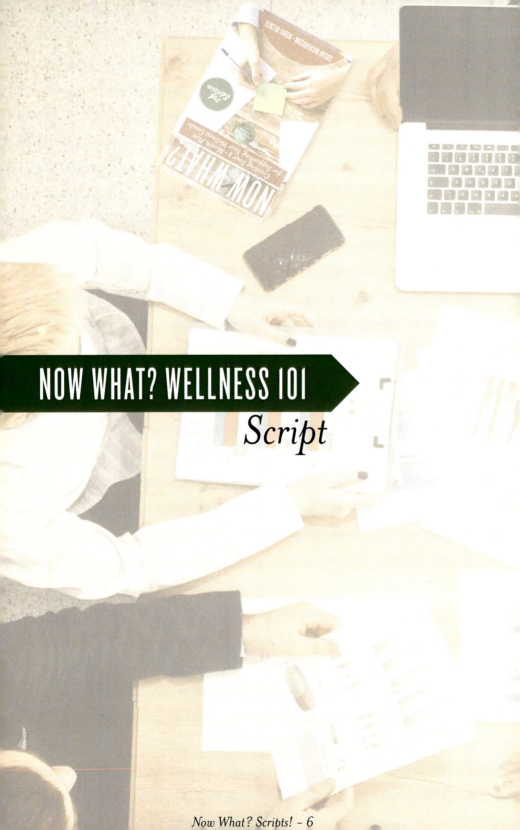

NOW WHAT? WELLNESS 101
Script

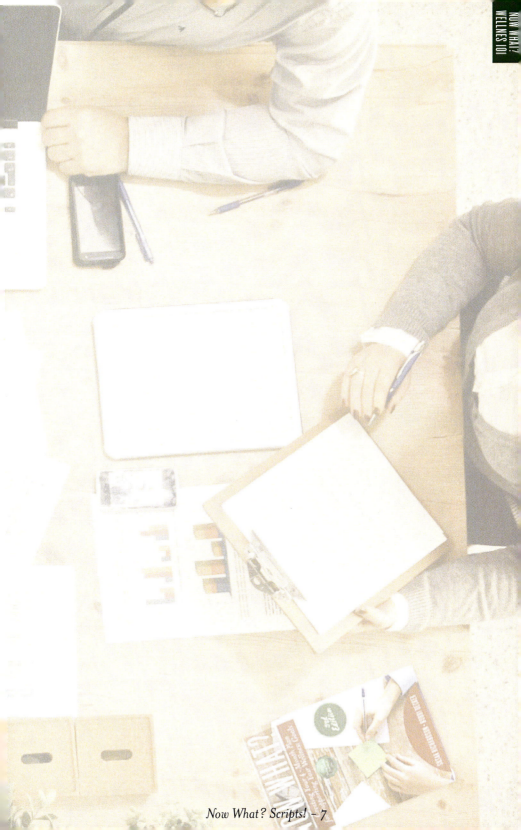

NOW WHAT? WELLNESS 101

Hi Everyone!! My name is _____ I'm a Young Living Brand Partner. First, I want to thank (Host/Hostess) for opening up his/her home to us so we can learn more about Young Living together. (Encourage host/hostess to briefly share their story.)

Did you know Young Living is actually a health and wellness company? (Pause, if they say no… say, most people don't and this is why _____ invited you.)

So, with this in mind, let's start by introducing ourselves and name one health goal that you have for you or a family member?

(Start with the person on your left… after each person tells you their health goal, hand them a Now What? book; and tell them which system of the body to bookmark and that you will explain why later. If you don't know the system of the body that is related to their goal, let them know that you will look that up and get back to them later in the class. Hand them a book and move on to the next person.)

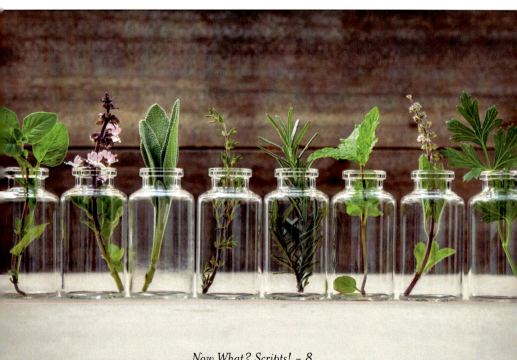

WHAT ARE ESSENTIAL OILS?

Essential oils are known as the lifeblood of the plant or the concentrated essence of the plant. They are volatile liquids and evaporate easily. Have you ever smelled the aroma of a plant? (Yes.) This means you have already safely experienced essential oils. These oils protect the plant from environmental stressors and disease. They also transport nutrients and oxygen throughout the plant. And, if they are properly grown and distilled, they do the same thing in your body.

To illustrate this, we are passing around Stress Away™. This is a blend of essential oils that works synergistically with each other and with your body. The name says it all. How many of you have experienced stress? EVERYONE, RIGHT!? Regardless of the source, a wedding, job interview or something more serious, stress is stress. You can even use it to replace perfumes or body sprays.

Another blend that benefits everyone is Peace & Calming. It's a blend that not only helps you relax, but a great choice for young children and pets. Just put a drop on your little one's feet or on your pet's ears and watch them settle right down.

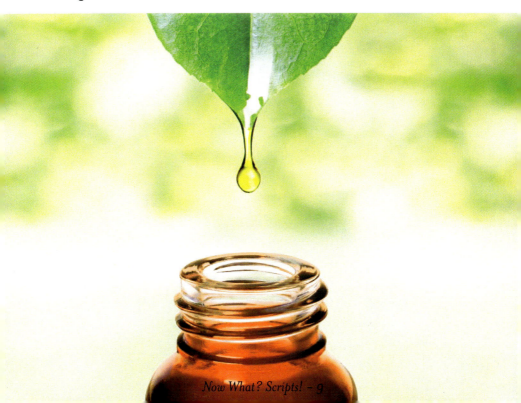

ESSENTIAL OIL HISTORY

Essential oils have been around since the beginning of time. They were mentioned in ancient scriptures and discovered in Egyptian tombs dating back more than 7,000 years. And even after all that time, these essential oils were found to still have an active phytochemical structure. While we don't expect to live to be 7,000 years old, this does tell us that if you store your premium essential oils properly, your essential oils will last indefinitely, too; they become a long-term investment. During ancient times, essential oils were thought to be more precious than gold.

Frankincense is considered a holy oil. But it is also one of the most versatile oils of modern times. It should be in everyone's home! Frankincense can be applied topically to help smooth the appearance of healthy looking skin. It can also slow the signs of aging on the skin, like liver spots and wrinkles. It is an excellent essential oil to use during massage, meditation, yoga, or prayer; and it is a key component of many essential oil blends that support mental acuity and focus. It can even help foster a positive outlook on life.

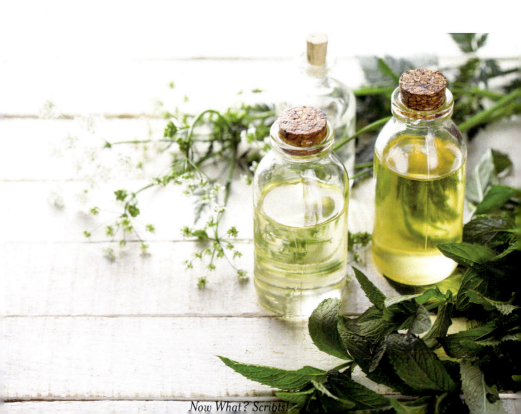

ALL ABOUT THIEVES

Another amazing thing essential oils do? They support the immune system. If you bookmarked the immune or respiratory system at the beginning of the class, pay attention to this.

There is an old legend, during the time of the plague, about four thieves that were walking among the dead and the dying and robbing them. The story goes that they never contracted the plague because they were oil and herb merchants who knew to rub the essential oils and spices of a plant on their bodies to offer protection. Isn't that fascinating?

Today, Young Living has a proprietary essential oil blend called Thieves. Thieves Vitality™ supports healthy immune and respiratory systems and protects our body's natural defenses. We can take this as a supplement in a gel cap or we can add it to a warm cup of water and honey. We use the classic blend to diffuse and purify our air or we rub it on the bottoms of our feet. (Share your personal Thieves story or ask the host/hostess to.)

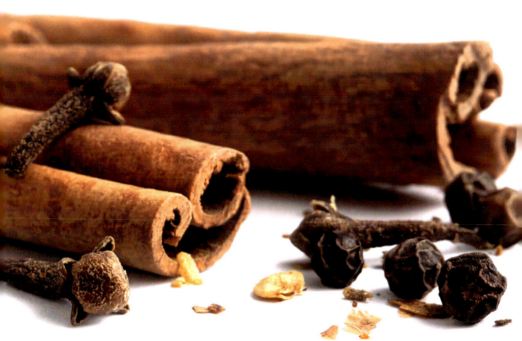

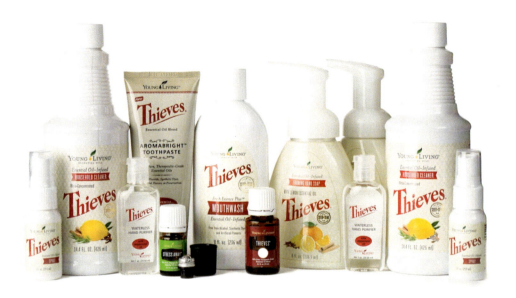

Because of the effectiveness of this blend, Young Living has an entire Thieves line. It includes items like household cleaner, hand soap, toothpaste, mouthwash, a misting spray, and even a waterless hand sanitizer that kills 99.99% of germs. I recommend that you keep this convenient item in your purse, backpack, diaper bag or desk. It is infused with thieves and peppermint essential oils, along with aloe to leave your hands not only clean, but soft without harsh chemicals found in other hand sanitizers.

Replace the harsh chemicals in your home with the Thieves Household Cleaner. Children, babies and pets are more vulnerable to chemical exposure because they are smaller, bioaccumulation happens more quickly and they aren't able to eliminate the toxins. Ditch those harsh chemicals and switch to a cleaner that is plant and mineral based so you can feel confident you are cleaning your home with absolute the best cleaner.

You can use this household cleaner on everything from lunch boxes to toilets. This plant based formula uses a naturally occurring surfactant derived from coconut and is non abrasive, leaves behind no chemical residue and is safe for septic systems. It is highly concentrated, making it cost effective! (Hold up pre-diluted spray bottle.) This bottle is my all-purpose cleaner. I add one cap of the Thieves Household Cleaner and fill the rest with water. I use this on everything.

By using these products, you will protect your home from harmful chemicals that can compromise your health while saving you money. And, it doesn't matter if you are brushing your teeth or scrubbing your toilet, you are supporting your health when you use any of the Thieves products.

NINGXIA RED

The first step toward any health goal, regardless of what system of the body you book-marked at the beginning of the class, is to make sure you fuel your body with dense nutrition! Meet NingXia Red (hold up bottle).

NingXia Red is a funny name, but NingXia is actually the name of a province in China where we get our wolfberries. The elderly in this community live to be centenarians. They contribute their longevity and health to the wolfberry which is full of dense nutrition. This wolfberry contains 4 times the nutrients than any other type of Goji berry from any other province, due to the volcanic ash and glacial runoff of that area.

There are actually 17 species of wolfberries, but ONLY the NingXia wolfberry has a complete phytonutrient profile. It is higher in vitamin C than oranges and higher in beta-carotene than carrots. It's also high in vitamin E and protein. It has amino acids, 21 trace minerals, 6 essential fatty acids, and vitamins B1, B2, & B6.

NingXia Red is a very high antioxidant puree, which means that it helps support our body's natural defense against aging. Dr. Richard Cutler of the National Institutes of Health said, "The amount of antioxidants that you maintain in your body is directly proportional to how long you live!"

The dense nutrition in this liquid supplement supports every system of the body, including the immune system (even our emotional well-being too). It contains high quality juices including blueberry, pomegranate, plum, cherry and aronia, but amazingly, even with these juices added, NingXia Red still supports normal blood sugar levels.

It offers cardiovascular support and protects normal liver and brain functions. There are no other products like NingXia Red on the market. NingXia Red is perfect for the person looking for whole body wellness, nutrition or just looking to maintain energy. energy. Who needs more energy? Let's do a Ningxia Shot.

NingXia Red and Thieves are the top two products in the company because they both help you accomplish your health goals, no matter what the goal.

It is super easy to integrate them into your daily routine by ordering them through Young Living's Subscribe to Save program. Just select the products you want, the frequency you want them, and have them shipped directly to your front door.

WHY YOUNG LIVING?

So, why would you want a to use Young Living's Subscribe to Save platform? Young Living is the only health and wellness company that has a Seed to Seal™ promise. This means Young Living oversees every step of the process, from the soil the seed is planted in to the sealed bottle that is delivered to your doorstep.

This is important because not all essential oils are created equally. Other companies may add synthetics, contaminants, and cheap fillers without regulation (even essential oils found on-line or in health food stores).

An essential oil only has to contain 10% essential oil to be labeled as an essential oil. BUT the alarming part is that according to the Federal Drug Administration's website, that 10% can be 100% synthetic. What does that mean? As long as a synthetic essential oil, like for instance Lavender, meets the chemical profile for the "actual lavender plant," it can be labeled exactly the same way. There is NO differentiation. But rest assured, there IS a difference and your body KNOWS.

When Young Living says its essential oils are premium, it means they are they have the highest standards in purity, potency, efficacy and quality. There are no synthetics, fillers, or harsh chemicals added to any of their essential oils or essential oil infused products. This is why it is important that you know your farmer, your distiller, and your source.

Young Living sources their vitality oils from plants grown from Non-GMO Project Verified seeds. To receive this certification, all Vitality oils must pass through a third-party verification, auditing, and testing process. (Canada also has a Non-GMO Project Verified certification on all its oils from the Plus(+) line.) This is yet another example of our Seed to Seal promise and commitment to the health and wellness of your family.

Young Living is also committed to ethical and sustainable production practices. Young Living gives back and improves the communities around the world where they have corporate-owned farms, partner farms, and Seed to Seal certified suppliers. Young Living even has a Foundation that serves these communities and proactively participates in global disaster relief. (If you have been to the YL Ecuador Academy or farm, share your experience here.)

Like the vitality essential oils, each batch of Young Living essential oil goes through a battery of tests. Young Living has in-house testing at the farms and at the labs around the world. Young Living routinely uses third party labs to ensure you get exactly what you expect, each and every time.

THE ABCS OF ESSENTIAL OIL USE

There are three ways you can use essential oils. You can **A**pply them, **B**reathe them, or **C**onsume them. To make this easy to remember, we call this the **ABCs** of essential oil use.

We can apply essential oils directly onto our skin or over an area that needs support. If you are using a "hot" oil, like Thieves, you will want to dilute it with a quality carrier oil like V-6. We also generally dilute oils when using with small children, the elderly, and pets. This slows down the rate of absorption.

We can breathe them in. We can put a drop of oil in the palm of our hand, rub our hands together, then cup them over our mouth and nose while taking several deep breaths. Some people like to do this to jump start their day or when life gets tough. Another way to get the aromatic benefits of essential oils is to use a diffuser like this one. *(Hold up a diffuser.) We can diffuse for calming, alerting, or purifying purposes. This is a simple yet strategic way to start implementing essential oils into your home.*

We can also consume essential oils. Young Living makes it easy to identify which oils can safely be taken as dietary supplements and/or used in the kitchen in place of spices, herbs, and citrus by labeling them as "Vitality Dietary Oils" -- the white label.

Young Living's essential oils and Vitality Oils are the exact same oil. The oils are equal in every way. They come from the same farms, from the same plants, and are bottled the same way. The only difference is the label.

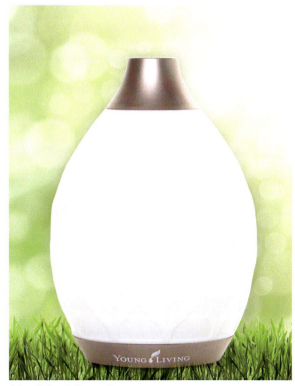

Now What? Scripts! – 15

EVERYDAY OILS

Lemon Vitality™ - is one of the most versatile of the Vitality Oils and is beneficial to virtually every system of your body. You can put several drops in a gel cap and take it as a dietary supplement. You can also add it to a glass of water or add flavor to your meals, like rice with chicken. The classic oil can be used to clean your white boards, to wipe down your counters, or for you moms, to help you remove gum from hair or stickers off walls.

Peppermint Vitality™ - as a dietary supplement, Peppermint Vitality can be used to support your digestive system and musculoskeletal system. Athletes love to infuse their water with Peppermint Vitality to help with stamina and endurance. You can also diffuse Peppermint for alertness and focus. And apply it topically on muscles after physical activity.

Joy - provides an aroma that brings joy to the heart, mind, and soul. You can use it as a perfume to help you with everyday blues and positivity. You can also add it to your diffuser to set the mood for a romantic evening with your partner.

Purification - is a blend that will help you ditch overpowering and harsh chemical-based sprays and keep your home smelling fresh and clean. Good Bye odors. We use this oil to eliminate bad odors from cooking, laundry, pets, or anything else life throws your way.

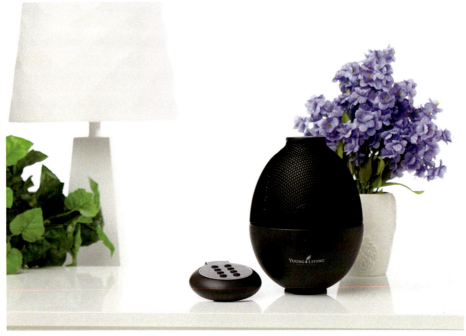

PanAway™ - is a classic oil formulated by D. Gary Young to soothe sore muscles after exercise. You can apply it to your wrists, back or head after sitting in a car or at a computer all day. This is an oil you may want to have extra of, to put in your purse or bag, so you have it where ever you go.

Valor - Many organizations award a Medal of Valor for physical courage. In fact, the Air Force's Medal of Honor displays the single word "Valor". This is an old-fashioned word that often describes warriors of the past and is the inspiration behind this blend… need a little courage? This is your oil. Diffuse it and apply it on your wrists and neck everyday for inner strength, fortitude and a greater sense of self. This is the first oil to be applied in Gary Young's Happy Day Protocol. When you get your first order, this should be the first oil you pull out and apply.

Tea Tree - is one of the most widely used and extensively researched essential oils, making it a must-have for every home. Because the benefits of Tea Tree include cleansing properties and a refreshing scent, this versatile oil can be used for everything from home cleaning solutions to skin care.

Lavender - is a one of the most versatile essential oils. It is often referred to as the "Swiss Army Knife" of essential oils. This is an oil you want in your home and on you at all times. You can diffuse it, apply it on your feet, or spray on your pillows for a restful night's sleep. Lavender is well known for its skin supporting properties. In fact, Young Living has an entire Lavender infused personal care line.

(Share your favorite personal care products here.)

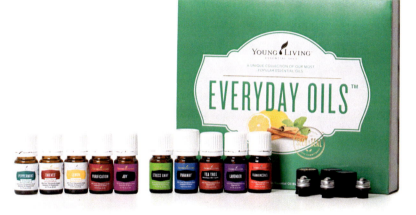

DID YOU KNOW?

Young Living has over 65 essential oil infused dietary supplements? How do you choose what's right for you? Well, YL makes it easy to identify their supplements! They come in three different colored labels: blue, green and red; and each has a very specific meaning in supporting your body.

The green labels are for foundational nutrition. This includes your multi-vitamins, probiotics, and minerals. These are the necessary nutrients that our bodies do not produce on their own, but need. If you are brand new to Young Living's supplements, the green ones are a great place to start. (Share your favorite foundational supplement.)

The blue labels are for cleansing. When you see a blue label we want you to remember digestive health and remember, all health begins in the gut. You will find many of these supplements in the Digestive chapter of your Now What? Book and Script book. (Share your favorite cleansing supplement.)

The red labels provide targeted nutrition for specific body systems and functions. Let's look at your Now What? Book. Turn to the body system you identified at the start of the class. Here you will discover which supplements will support your health goal best. (Share your favorite targeted nutrition supplement.)

So, we have covered a lot of information. YL has over 600 products for your home, beauty and health. So how do you know what to choose?

First, understand you have us! We are your support team; we will lock arms with you and help you every step of the way. Getting Young Living into your home is the first step, it's simple and were here to help you get started. The average American household spends about $150 per month on personal care items, cleaning supplies and supplements. We will teach you how to take the money you already spend on your makeup, all purpose cleaners, toothpaste, hand sanitizers, vitamins, etc. And transfer it to Young Living's shopping platform.

Once you create your account you can easily log in, add these items to your Subscribe to Save cart, decide how frequent you want them (every month, every 2 or even 3 months) and have them delivered straight to your door just like you do on Amazon or other shopping sites you trust and love. And the best part? By being a Subscribe to Save customer you will unlock Young Living's 24% discount on every item you order as long as you keep something on your Subscribe to Save cart.

NOW WHAT?

The other option is to focus more on your health goal first and use your Now What? Book to create your 4-Month Wellness plan. If you did not choose a health goal, you can turn to the Maintaining System Health plan. Check off the products you want and use that as a guide to set up your Subscribe to Save cart.

(Ask the guests to pull out their smartphones or tablet and log into the Young Living Website. You can also send the guests a link to the My YL Bundle that corresponds with their health goal. Help them navigate the shopping platform and create their account.)
Now What?

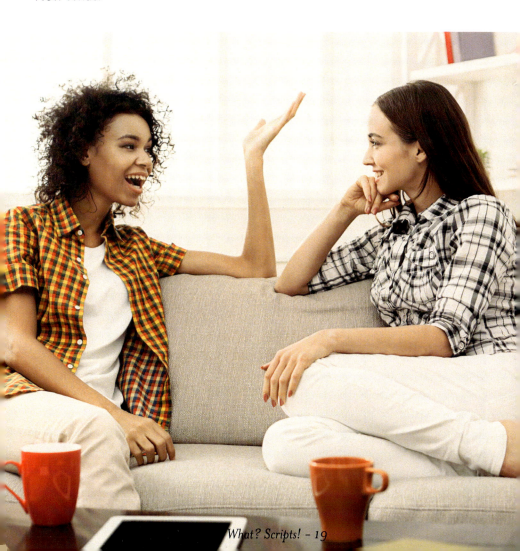

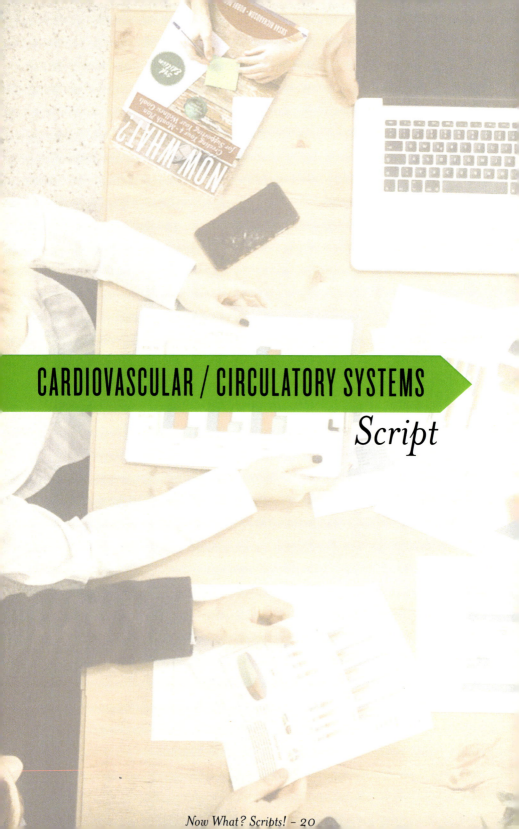

CARDIOVASCULAR / CIRCULATORY SYSTEMS
Script

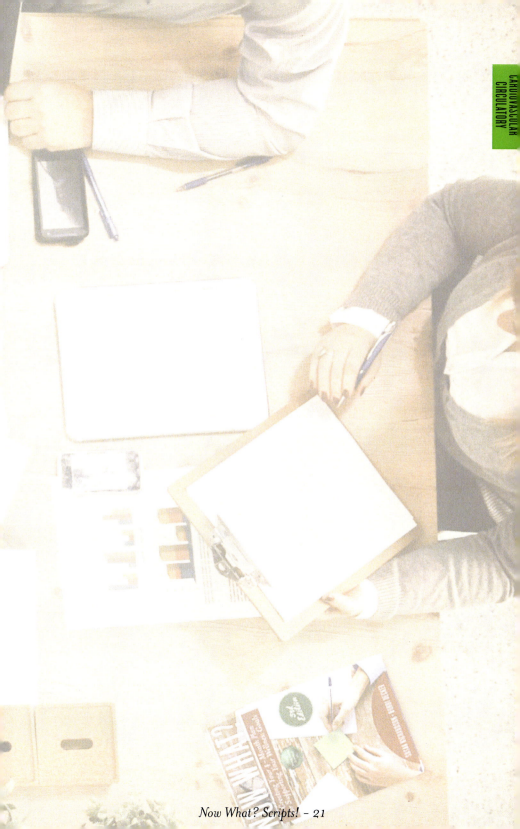

CARDIOVASCULAR / CIRCULATORY SYSTEM

Hello everyone, in case you don't know me, my name is _____ . I am part of your Young Living Support Team. Thank you for being a part of our oily family. I want to thank (Hostess/Host) for opening up his/her home to us, so we can learn more about how to take your health to the next level.

As Young Living customers, we all know what essential oils are and how they work in our bodies. Essential oils and essential oil-infused products are the number one way to protect your home from harsh chemicals and toxins; and promote health for you and your entire family.

Because Young Living is a health and wellness company, we are able to address wellness from a whole body perspective. And, we can also look more in-depth at individual body systems like we are going to do today with the cardiovascular system.

This shouldn't shock you, but we discourage people from buying just a single oil. However, if that is what you choose, we recommend you put it on a Subscribe to Save oder to help you save money. We don't want to mislead you into thinking that using just one bottle of oil is going to achieve your health goals. Instead, we like to empower you with healthy lifestyle habits and with help to set up your own 4-Month Wellness Plan so you can reach and maintain your health goals.

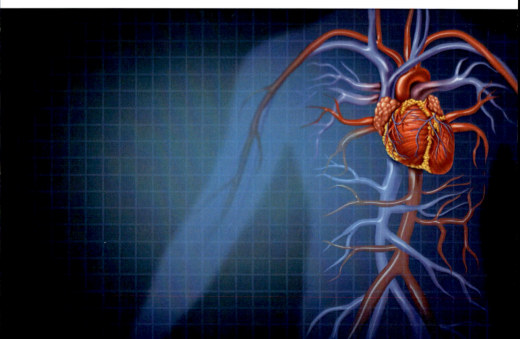

Young Living makes it easy to get these products into your home through the Subscribe to Save shopping platform. If you are not familiar with this yet, you are going to be SO happy!!

With all this in mind, let's take a closer look at the cardiovascular system and discuss a few ways to address this system of the body so you can keep it above the health line.

Open your Now What? book to the cardiovascular system on page 8. This system circulates the blood around the body via the heart, veins, and arteries. This oxygenates the cells in your body, delivers nutrients, and carries away waste products. The heart is the body's hardest working organ, so let's make sure we do what we need to do to take care of it.

Do you have a mediocre diet? (Wait for a yes.)
Have you ever been so busy that you forgot to eat a meal? (Wait for a yes.)

This isn't good for your heart, which is why it is SO important to do everything you can to ensure you and your family are getting the proper nutrition you need to support every system of your body.

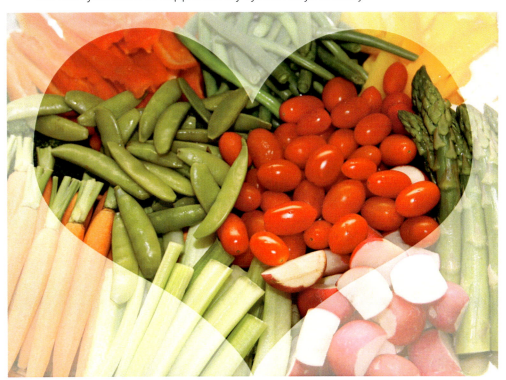

We know that when we use an essential oil-infused product, it helps our body absorb and distribute nutrition from the foods we eat and makes the nutrients from our supplements we take more bioavailable. We can even use the Vitality essential oils as dietary supplements. You should already have some Vitality Dietary Essential Oils and Classic Essential Oils. Whatever you have, make sure you pull them out and use them every day.

Cinnamon Bark is also well known for supporting heart health. Young Living's Cinnamon Bark Vitality is an easy way to get the constituents of this spice into our bodies. You can easily add a drop of Cinnamon and Orange Vitality to your morning NingXia Red shot to support your cardio system every morning.

Let's all do a NingXia shot while we discuss NingXia Red. **(Pass cardio shots around.)**

NingXia Red supports every system of the body, even for those of us who are already healthy. NingXia Red helps us to maintain that health, stamina, and cognitive wellness. Today we are going to focus on how the ingredients in NingXia Red support cardiovascular health.

It is a funny name, but NingXia is actually the name of the province in China where the primary ingredient is grown. The NingXia wolfberry is the predominant food of the people in this region who live to be over 100 years old. They contribute their health and longevity to this particular wolfberry which is packed full of dense nutrition and contains 4x the nutrients of the wolfberries in neighboring provinces.

NingXia Red is very high in antioxidants, which means that it helps support our body's natural defense against aging. Dr. Richard Cutler, National Institutes of Health said, "The amount of antioxidants that you maintain in your body is directly proportional to how long you live!"

In addition, antioxidants have been evaluated for both primary and secondary support of your cardiovascular system.

There are actually 17 species of wolfberry and only the NingXia wolfberry has a complete phytonutrient profile. It is higher in vitamin C than oranges, higher in betacarotene than carrots and higher in calcium than cauliflower.

Calcium is responsible for functions in the body like regulating normal blood pressure. There is solid evidence that indicates calcium is necessary for proper health.

NingXia Red is also high in vitamin E and protein. NingXia Wolfberries are a good source of amino acids and 21 trace minerals which are important for all of the body systems to properly function.

NingXia Wolfberries also have 6 essential fatty acids which is important because our body cannot make essential fatty acids, they must come from our diet.

NingXia Red has vitamins B1, B2, & B6 and more. This is dense nutrition. And let's face it, most people are not getting what they need from the food they eat.

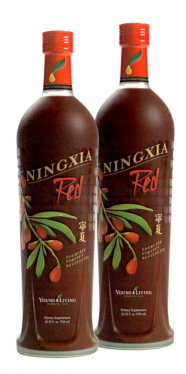

It contains high quality juices and purees including blueberry, pomegranate, plum, and cherry. Amazingly, even with these juices included, it still supports healthy blood sugar levels and offers low glycemic energy. This is because it is a puree and contains the fruit fiber.

NingXia Red contains a patented grape seed extract that contains polyphenolic compounds that may help support a healthy cardiovascular system as well.

Another thing that sets NingXia Red apart is that it is the only nutritive supplement available that is infused with essential oils. This aids the body's ability to absorb and assimilate all of those nutrients offering whole body support including our ability to cope with stress.

Let's talk a little bit about physical activity because while diet and nutrition are important, it's good to move your body. The American Heart Association recommends for a healthy heart to get 150 minutes of moderate exercise a week. Being physically active is important in preventing heart disease and stroke. Just 30 minutes of walking a day will decrease your chances of falling below the heart health line. So, let's all stand up and move. Change seats and sit by someone new. Seriously, let's get up and move.

4-MONTH WELLNESS PLAN

We have discussed NingXia Red and the fact that it is the foundation for every system, so it stands to reason that it is the first addition to your 4-Month Wellness Plan. It doesn't matter what your goal is, this is our #1 choice for everyone. Let's also talk about MindWise. This is an AMAZING supplement that everyone should be taking along with their NingXia Red. The MindWise proprietary memory blend features ALCAR (acetyl-L-carnitine). This functions as an antioxidant and promotes the production of glutathione and is a free radical scavenger.

MindWise™ also has glycerophosphocholine or GPC, a natural physiological precursor to a neurotransmitter that is involved in memory and other cognitive functions and is known to cross the blood brain barrier. Clinical studies have demonstrated it helps to support cognitive function and mental acuity. MindWise™ also contains medium chain triglycerides (MCT) from coconut oil and generous amounts of vitamin D3; both promote cardiovascular health.

CoQ10 is found in every cell of the body and is necessary for the basic functioning of cells and has been studied for supporting healthy brain function. CoQ10 supplementation has also been documented to show sustained cholesterol levels, circulatory function, and normal overall heart and cardiovascular health.

Another supplement and great complimentary product also combining Vitamin D3, CoQ10 and fatty acids is OmegaGize3, which is infused with DHA-rich fish oil and essential oils which work synergistically to support normal brain, heart, eye, and joint health.

CardioGize is an herbal supplement infused with essential oils that has a synergistic ratio of CoQ10 and selenium as well as vitamin K, garlic and more. CardioGize supports the entire vascular system including proper blood circulation.

There are thousands of research articles published on the health benefits of garlic alone. It has been documented that garlic supports the body's natural response to artery plaque formation and blood stickiness and helps to maintain healthy blood pressure levels, triglycerides and blood glucose levels.

Studies have also shown that by combining CoQ10 and selenium in the proper ratio helps to protect our heart from oxidative stress, reducing cardiac incidents. Other studies have revealed that Vitamin K is directly correlated to heart health. And while eating your green leafy vegetables is a good start, supplementation may be beneficial in promoting heart, brain and musculoskeletal health.

The CardioGize supplement was made possible by the dedicated research and work of our late founder, D. Gary Young. Before his passing, he described the process behind the creation of this product, saying: "After testing to determine various compounds, I put the formula together for the most synergic, powerful, and beneficial response for the body."

Good Nutrition is tied to good health and while we get many of our nutrients from food, sometimes supplementation is necessary, like with our B vitamins. Super B is a comprehensive vitamin complex containing all eight essential, bioavailable energy-boosting B vitamins (B1, B2, B3, B5, B6, B7, B9, and B12). The body needs these B vitamins for all of the systems of the body to function properly, but also to nurture the cardiovascular system by promoting the production of red blood cells and to support the body's ability to effectively and naturally deal with sticky blood.

Longevity Softgels™ are a dietary supplement containing fractionated coconut oil along with a blend of Thyme, Clove, Frankincense and Orange essential oils. We can take this supplement daily to strengthen the body's systems to safeguard against the damaging effects of aging, diet, and the environment.

While supplements and Vitality Oils offer targeted system support, the "You May Also Like" products are a great addition to your 4-Month Wellness Plan. One such essential oil blend you may enjoy for a calming and de-stressing effect is Aroma Life. You can wear this blend topically over your heart center or on your forearms, or put it in your diffuser for a relaxing aroma.

Ylang Ylang is another perfect complementary product for your cardiovascular 4-Month Wellness Plan. With its sweet aroma, it will help support positive emotions, mood, and energy levels. Studies have shown the inhalation of Ylang Ylang for 20 minutes - use your diffusers - and the topical application to the abdomen show a correlation in sustaining heart health.

The products we covered today are great examples of what you can put on your Subscribe to Save order to jump start your 4-Month Wellness Plan. But remember, everybody is different. Sometimes we have an immediate response using Young Living products. I am sure we all can agree that one drop of oil will not really support the underlying signals your body may be giving you. You need to make a commitment to use your products consistently. Be okay with that.

You've already started by being here. Now use your NOW WHAT? book to set up a 4-Month Wellness Plan. Check off the products you want to order each month on page 9.

And remember to personalize your choices. Look at the "You May Also Like" Products and choose from there, too. If you are personalizing for a child, you may want to incorporate the KidScents™ products on page 43. If you want to take it up a notch, you may want to incorporate the cardio Raindrop products on page xx.

(Give the guests a few minutes to develop their plan. Be available to help them personalize, otherwise, sit back, be quiet and let them think.)

Okay, now that you all have your plan, pull out your smartphone and log into onto your shopping platform. We are going to set up your first month's order with Subscribe to Save. If you are not familiar with this yet, this will save you money while getting the products you need to get well. Remember, if you order more than 50pv you will earn free products through our Loyalty Rewards program too. All you have to do is make sure you consistently process 50pv every month to participate.

I have your member number if you don't know it. (Coach them through setting up their orders. You can send the guests a link to the My YL Bundle that corresponds with their health goal. Help them navigate the shopping platform and create their account.)

CARDIOVASCULAR
CIRCULATORY

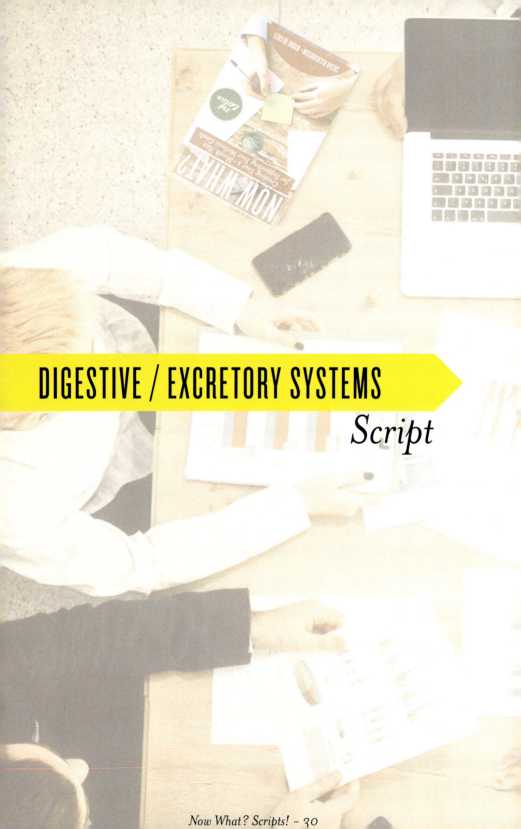

DIGESTIVE / EXCRETORY SYSTEMS
Script

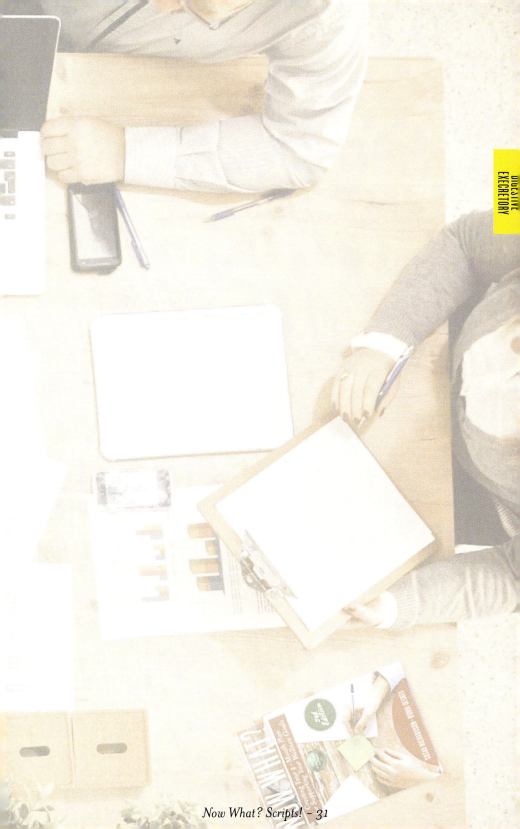

DIGESTIVE / EXCRETORY SYSTEM

Hello everyone, in case you don't know me, my name is _____ . I am part of your Young Living Support Team. Thank you for being a part of our oily family. I want to thank *(Hostess)* for opening up his/her home to us so we can learn more about how to take your health to the next level.

As Young Living customers, we all know what essential oils are and how they work in our bodies. Essential oils and essential oil-infused products are the number one way to protect your home from harsh chemicals and toxins; and promote health for you and your entire family.

Because Young Living is a health and wellness company, we are able to address wellness from a whole body perspective. And we can also look more in-depth at individual body systems, like we are going to do today with the Digestive System.

This shouldn't shock you, but we discourage people from buying just a single oil. However, if that is what you choose, we recommend you put it on a Subscribe to Save oder to help you save money. We don't want to mislead anyone into thinking one bottle of oil can help them achieve their health goals. Instead, we like to empower you with healthy lifestyle habits and to set up your own 4-Month Wellness Plan so you can reach and maintain your health goals.

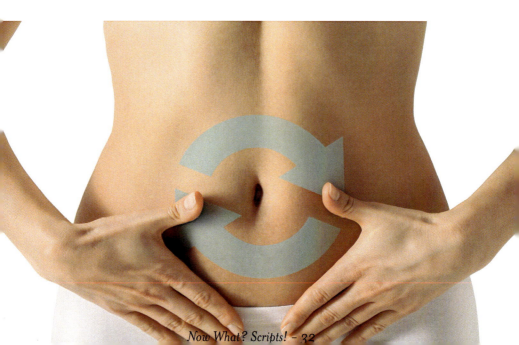

With all this in mind, let's take a closer look at the digestive system and discuss a few ways to address this system of the body so you can keep it above the health line.

Open your Now What? book to the Digestive System on page 10. This system consists of the mechanical and chemical processes that deliver nutrients to our body and eliminate waste. These processes allow the body to produce energy and maintain normal cell function. Who wants more energy?

Remember all health begins in the digestive system, so let's make sure we do what we need to do to give it what it needs to take care of us.

Most of us know that the bacteria in our gut play an important role in digestion. If you didn't know that… surprise, you have good bacteria in your gut working to help you. When the digestive system struggles to digest the food we eat, more gut microbes jump in to offer a helping hand, ensuring we are able to properly assimilate the nutrients we need. In addition, gut bacteria are known to aid the production of certain vitamins - such as vitamins B and K - and play a major role in immune function.

Two-thirds of this gut microbiome is unique to each person. This is because our microbiome is determined by the foods we eat, the air we breathe, and other environmental factors such as the pollutants we breathe from smog and chemical cleaners to the products we put on our bodies like lotions, makeup, soaps, shampoos and conditioners. Who knew the makeup or personal care products you use every day were potentially toxic to your digestive system?

It's true, and an unhealthy digestive terrain has been linked to so many other health issues. By taking care of your digestive system, you are giving your body what it needs to properly take care of itself and stay ABOVE the health line.

Do you have a mediocre diet? *(Wait for a yes.)*
Have you ever been so busy that you forgot to eat a meal? *(Wait for a yes.)*

This isn't good for your gut, which is why it is SO important to do everything you can to ensure you and your family are getting the proper nutrition you need to support every system of your body AND that your body is able to utilize it.

We know that when we use an essential oil-infused product, it helps our body absorb nutrition from the foods we eat and makes the nutrients from our supplements we take more bioavailable. You should already have some Vitality oils and Classic Essential Oils. Whatever you have, make sure you pull them out and use them every day. We recommend you get Peppermint, DiGize and Lemon Vitality, if you don't already have them.

Another way to get the benefits of lemon is through organic whole lemon powder in AlkaLime. AlkaLime neutralizes acidity and stabilizes pH levels to maintain not only gut health, but overall health and energy as well. You can take this product one hour before meals or bed time.

Young Living is a company that strives to focus on nutrition and all that is good for you. They have a wide range of ways to help you meet your goals. JuvaPower® is a high antioxidant vegetable powder complex and is one of the richest sources of acid-binding foods. It also helps to support the healthy function of the Digestive System with a focus on the liver. You even open up the capsule and sprinkle it over your food like salads, chicken or potatoes. You can even add it to your juice or even give it to your pets. Just sprinkle a little over their food and call it a day.

The foods we eat today lack the nutrients and enzymes our body needs. Allerzyme is a powerful vegetarian enzyme supplement that aids digestion and relieves bloating and gas. Allerzyme may reduce food-related discomfort. Who's excited about that?

One way to ensure you are getting your nutrients, fiber, minerals, and protein is by using our amazing Balance Complete. Not only is it a great meal replacement, but along with Ningxia Red, it is a key component of our nutritive cleanse. Everyone needs a good cleansing. The 5 day nutritive cleanse is very gentle and nourishing. The Cleansing Trio is targeted towards the elimination of waste and enhancing proper liver function. When

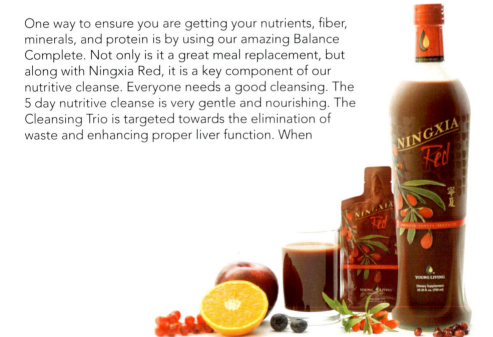

our gut and liver are cleansed properly we can absorb even more nutrition which will affect overall wellbeing. This is an important step to systemic health.

We also have Tangerine Vitality which is well known for supporting digestive health too. Young Living's Tangerine Vitality is an easy way to get the constituents of this fruit's rind. You can easily add a drop of Tangerine and Fennel Vitality to your morning NingXia Red shot to support your digestive system every morning.

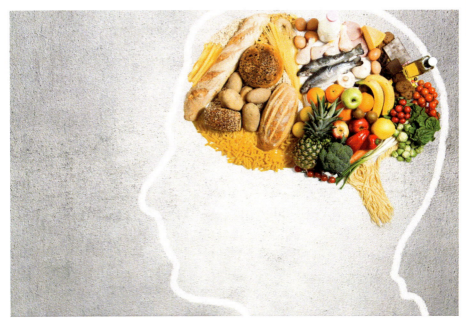

Let's all do a NingXia Shot while we discuss NingXia Red and digestive health. *(Pass Digestive shots around.)*

NingXia Red is a supplement that we should actually be drinking daily. We recommend that this be the first thing you put on your 4-Month Wellness Plan because NingXia Red supports the Digestive System as well as every other system of the body. Even for those of us who are already healthy, NingXia Red helps us to maintain that health, stamina, and cognitive wellness.

It is a funny name, but NingXia is actually the name of the province in China where the primary ingredient is grown. The NingXia Wolfberry is the predominant food of the people in this region who live to be over 100 years old. They contribute their health and longevity to this particular wolfberry which is packed full of dense nutrition and contains 4x the nutrients of the wolfberries in neighboring provinces and scores 3290 on the ORAC scale.

If you aren't familiar with the ORAC scale, the bottom line is that the score measures the antioxidant capacity of a food. The higher the number, the better/more effective it is. Antioxidants give the lining of the gut TLC and protect the cells by naturally keeping inflammation at bay. They also promote the growth of good bacteria.

Dr. Richard Cutler, National Institutes of Health said, "The amount of antioxidants that you maintain in your body is directly proportional to how long you live!"

There are actually 17 species of wolfberry and only the NingXia Wolfberry has a complete phyto-nutrient profile. It is higher in vitamin C than oranges, higher in calcium than cauliflower, and higher in beta-carotene than carrots. It's also high in vitamin E and protein.

It is rich in amino acids like L-glutamine which is important for healthy gut function.

NingXia Red contains 21 trace minerals which are important for all of the body systems to properly function, 6 essential fatty acids that help the body naturally respond to normal gut inflammation, and even vitamins B1, B2, and B6, which help your body change the carbohydrates in your diet into energy for your cells and keep your appetite regulated.

This is dense nutrition. And let's face it, most people are not getting what they need from the food they eat.

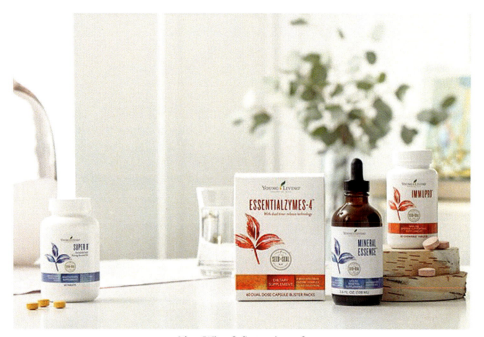

NingXia Red also contains high quality juices and purees like blueberry, pomegranate, plum, and cherry. Amazingly, even with these juices included, it still supports healthy blood sugar levels. This is because it is a puree and contains the fruit fiber.

Another thing that sets NingXia Red apart is that it is the only nutritive supplement available that is infused with essential oils. This aids the body's ability to absorb, distribute and assimilate all of those nutrients offering crucial digestive support.

Let's talk a little bit about physical activity because while diet and nutrition are important, it's also good to move your body. The American Heart Association recommends for a healthy heart you need to get 150 minutes of moderate exercise a week. Research also has shown that exercise can help with occasional gas or bloating, and that physical movement and activity can help to stimulate movement of the bowels. Just 30 minutes of walking a day can decrease your chances of falling below the health line. So as an exercise in movement, let's all stand up and exchange seats… sit next to someone different. Okay, let's do it.

We have discussed NingXia Red and that it is the foundation for every system, so it stands to reason that it is the first addition to your 4-Month Wellness Plan. It doesn't matter what your goal is, this is our #1 choice for everyone.

As we know, all health begins in the digestive system. Along with NingXia Red, Digize Vitality is a great companion supplement to use with every meal to promote proper digestion. We can also use it when traveling abroad, on airplanes and boats, and for occasional tummy upsets. You can also put a drop or two in a gel cap and take internally as a dietary supplement for gastrointestinal support.

Did you know that 70% of your Immune System stems from the Digestive System? Billions of microorganisms live in our Digestive System. Master Formula and ICP Daily contain prebiotics. You've heard of PRO-biotics as being healthy gut flora or "good bacteria." Well, PRE-biotics feed that good bacteria allowing the immune cells to work throughout the body without having to focus on the Digestive System. So, when you add Master Formula and ICP Daily to your wellness plan, you are providing even more gut health, AND, as a side effect, a healthy gut means stronger immune system. Antioxidants plus prebiotics means a stronger immune and digestive support.

When we take care of our microbiome, the benefits are vast. It will give us the ability to stay active, sustain energy, and promote nutrient absorption such as folate (needed for healthy cell reproduction), B12 helps make DNA and red blood cells, and fatty acids which help maintain healthy cells in the bowel wall.

> *Young Living doesn't create its oils in a lab. In fact, it is the only Health and Wellness company in the WORLD which owns its own farms and distilleries and produces the most premium essential oils and essential oil-infused products.*
>
> *Anyone can go to a Young Living Farm to experience and participate in the farming, distilling and testing practices first hand.*

When Young Living says its essential oils are premium, it means they have the highest standards in purity, potency, efficacy and quality. There are no synthetics, fillers, or harsh chemicals added to any of their essential oils or essential oil infused products.

When looking to balance the health of the Digestive System, along with Sulfurzyme, Young Living took the guesswork out with the dynamic duo of Inner Defense and Life 9. Inner Defense is basically Thieves Vitality in a capsule combined with the proper ratio of Thyme Vitality, Oregano Vitality and Lemongrass Vitality for extra support. Inner Defense creates an unfriendly terrain for yeast and fungus in your gut. It tends to be most effective when taken 6-8 hours before our probiotic, Life 9. Life 9 is pretty amazing because it has 9 clinically proven high-potency probiotic strains that do not inhibit each other. It combines 17 billion live cultures from these 9 bacteria strains that promote healthy digestion, gut health and helps maintain normal intestinal function.

4-MONTH WELLNESS PLAN

The products we covered today are great examples of what you can put on your Subscribe to Save order to jump start your 4-Month Wellness Plan. But remember, everybody is different. While sometimes we have an immediate response using Young Living products, I am sure we all can agree that one drop of oil will not really support the underlying signals your body may be giving you. You need to make a commitment to use your products consistently. Be okay with that.

You've already started by being here. Now use your NOW WHAT? book to set up a 4-Month Wellness Plan. Check off the products you want to order each month on page 11.

Remember to personalize your choices. Look at the "You May Also Like" Products and choose from there, too. If you are personalizing for a child, you may want to incorporate the Kidscents products on page 51. If you want to take it up a notch, you may want to incorporate the Digestive Raindrop products. (see page 44).

(Give the guests a few minutes to develop their plan. Be available to help them personalize, otherwise, sit back, be quiet and let them think.)

Okay, now that you all have your plan, pull out your smartphone and log onto your Subscribe to Save. If you are not familiar with this yet, this will save you money while getting the products you need to get well. Remember, if you order more than 50pv you will earn free products through our Loyalty Rewards program too. All you have to do is make sure you consistently process 50pv every month to participate.

We are going to set up your first month's order with Subscribe and Save. I have your member number if you don't know it. *(Coach them through setting up their order. You can send the guests a link to the My YL Bundle that corresponds with their health goal. Help them navigate the shopping platform and create their account.)*

> *While sometimes, we have an immediate response using Young Living products. I am sure we all can agree that one drop of oil will not really support the underlying signals your body may be giving you. You will need to make a commitment to use your products consistently. Be okay with that. We recommend you start by getting the wholesale membership, then use your NOW WHAT? book to set up a 4-Month Wellness Plan and set up your first month on Essential Rewards.*

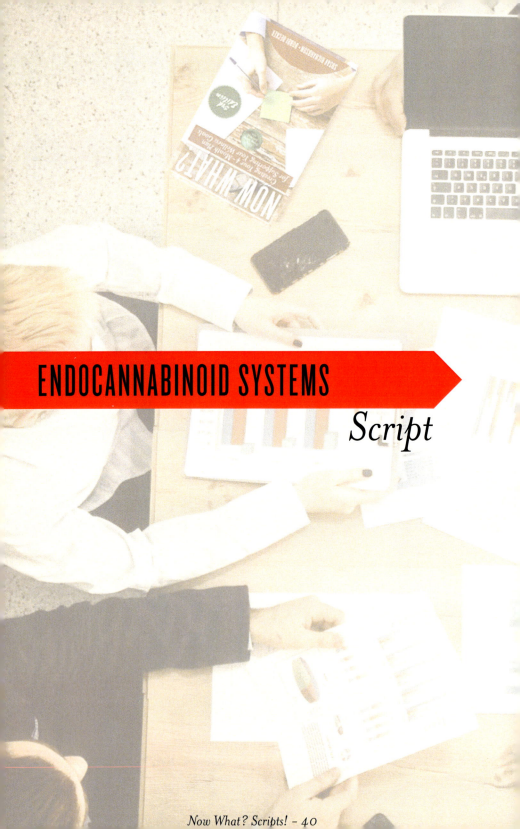

ENDOCANNABINOID SYSTEMS

Script

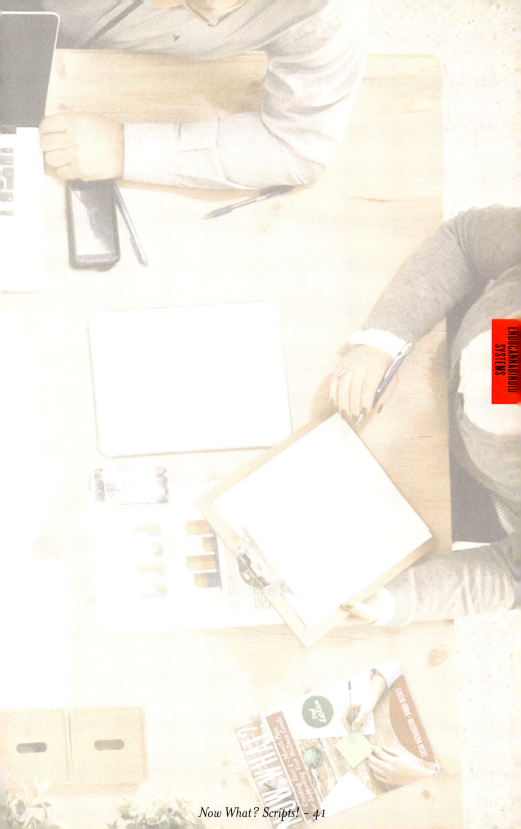

ENDOCANNABINOID SYSTEM

Hello everyone, in case you don't know me, my name is _____ . I am part of your Young Living Support Team. Thank you for being a part of our oily family. I want to thank (Hostess/Host) for opening up his/her home to us, so we can learn more about how to take your health to the next level.

As Young Living customers, we all know what essential oils are and how they work in our bodies. Essential oils and essential oil-infused products are the number one way to protect your home from harsh chemicals and toxins; and promote health for you and your entire family.

Because Young Living is a health and wellness company, we are able to address wellness from a whole body perspective. And we can also look more in-depth at individual body systems like we are going to do today with the endocannabinoid system.

This shouldn't shock you, but we discourage people from buying just a single oil. However, if that is what you choose, we recommend you put it on your Subscribe to Save order to help save money. We don't want to mislead anyone into thinking one bottle of oil can achieve your health goals. Instead, we like to empower you with healthy lifestyle habits and to set up your own 4-Month Wellness Plan so you can reach and maintain your health goals.

With all this in mind, let's take a closer look at the endocannabinoid system and discuss a few ways to address this system so you can stay above the health line.

Open your Now What? book to the endocannabinoid system on page 12. This system was discovered in the early 1990s. It is a group of specific membrane receptors that are located in the brain and throughout the central and peripheral nervous system. The endocannabinoid system acts as a relay switch from your brain to the rest of your body. If this switch is broken or compromised, your brain cannot communicate with the other body systems.

You may have heard of the presence of cannabinoids in cannabis, which are found in everything from marijuana seeds to CBD oil, but you might not know how they can help you. Fortunately, because our endocannabinoid system (ECS) regulates functions like our appetite, memory, mood, nerve and immune function, the CBD oil can be used to assist in balancing the body. This is because plant cannabinoids work to stimulate the body and bind to receptors. So, the goal, no matter what is being addressed is always the same: bringing the body back to homeostasis. And when we have homeostasis we are healthy.

We want you to understand that everyone already has naturally occurring cannabinoids (CBD) in their body. According to the findings of several major scientific studies, human breast milk contains the same cannabinoids found in the cannabis plant. In fact, every cell in our body produces cannabinoids and they are vital for proper human development.

You already know that hemp has cannabinoids, but did you know that cannabinoids are in many of the plants we consume everyday? This includes clove, black pepper, echinacea, broccoli, ginseng and carrots. We obviously don't get a high from eating our broccoli and drinking our tea. That is because CBD is different from THC. The CBD does not interact with the body the same way the THC does; there are no psychoactive properties in CBD, so there are no euphoric feelings or altered mental states.

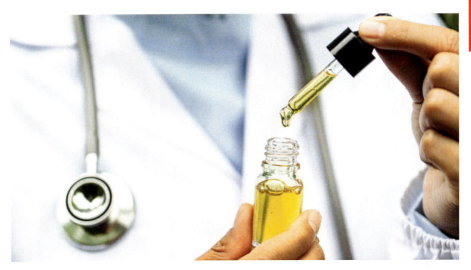

How Does this work?

Simply put, CBD isolate is the cannabinoid in its purest form. CBD isolate crystals contain JUST that chemical compound... CBD... That's it, No THC, No terpenes, just cannabinoids. This is why Nature's Ultra CBD will not get you high or show up on a drug test; this is also how essential oils come into play.

The CBD isolate is inert. But, when a terpene rich premium essential oil like Young Living's is added to the CBD isolate, the essential oil activates the CBD with naturally occurring terpenes. This makes both the essential oil and CBD work better. In fact, this makes it even more effective than full spectrum CBD.

There are specific terpenes found in the essential oils that optimize the outcome of the CBD, so Young Living partnered with Nature's Ultra to formulate easy to use CBD products. You can choose from these products based on the aroma of the essential oil it is infused with or you can choose based on the essential oil compounds.

Those of us who already use Young Living Essential Oils, know that plants play a key part in our health. Copaiba is the most concentrated source of the terpene ß-caryophyllene you'll find in the plant world. So by adding a drop of Copaiba or even other terpene rich oils like Black Pepper, Orange, Clove, Rosemary, Oregano, Basil, Lavender, or Cinnamon Bark vitality oil to your morning NingXia Red shot, you are giving your endocannabinoid system an excellent sources of ß-caryophyllene. When paired with any one of our CBD products you are supporting your ECS in a profound way.

Just like CBD, NingXia Red supports every system of the body. It also has cherry juice in the formula which contains anthocyanins that interact at the cannabinoid receptor sites. This flavonoid is known to support your body's healthy response to everyday pain and inflammation. NingXia Red is Young Living's Antioxidant supplement. When the endocannabinoid is paired with antioxidants, it protects against cell damage promoting healthy cell function throughout the body. This includes how it affects your heart, kidneys, brain, other organs and body systems. This makes CBD and NingXia Red an impressive combination that helps the expression of health throughout the body. (See the other Now What scripts for more information for additional Ningxia Red benefits.)

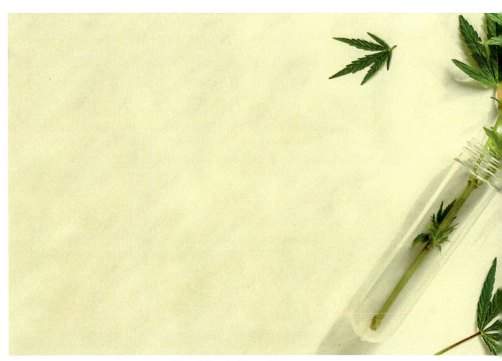

We have discussed NingXia Red and the fact that it is the foundation for every system, so it stands to reason that it is the first addition to your 4-Month Wellness Plan. It doesn't matter what your goal is, this is our #1 choice for everyone. Let's also talk about MindWise. This is an AMAZING supplement that everyone should be taking along with their NingXia Red. Like NingXia Red, this functions as an antioxidant and promotes the production of glutathione and is a free radical scavenger.

MindWise™ contains glycerophosphocholine (GPC), a natural precursor to a neurotransmitter that is involved in memory, other cognitive functions and is known to cross the blood brain barrier. Like GPC, CBD has many well documented neuroprotective properties. MindWise contains medium chain triglycerides (MCT) from coconut oil which helps make the CBD more bioavailable.

CoQ10, found in MindWise, is a fat soluble antioxidant which is found in every cell of the body and is necessary for the basic functioning of cells. Studies have also shown that CoQ10 supplementation may be beneficial in assisting the ECS in promoting heart, brain and musculoskeletal health.

Another great supplement to support the endocannabinoid system is OmegaGize3. This combines Vitamin D3, CoQ10 and other essential fatty acids , which is infused with DHA-rich fish oil and essential oils.

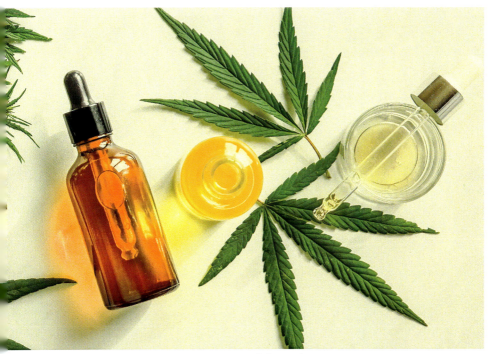

Now What? Scripts!

The Omega 3's are the building blocks for endocannabinoids and help stabilize the function of the ECS. They have been shown to help with people who experience the everyday blues, anxiousness, and who need a little extra mood support.

Have you ever heard of the brain - gut connection? It's true, it's a thing. And to be more precise, your gut has a brain. This second brain won't help you math or remember a password, but its connection to the brain in your head plays a major role in everything we are talking about.

Many researchers believe the ECS is the communication link between the gut and the brain that enables them to "speak" to each other.

Remember when we said the ECS acts as a relay switch? The ECS regulates the two-way communication between the gut and the brain. Changes in the brain related to stress or pain can alter gastrointestinal function. In addition, changes in your gut from inflammation or infection are communicated back to the brain via the ECS. This is important in maintaining bowel health and can even influence conditions like irritable bowel syndrome.

How can you support your ECS for a healthy gut? First, we need to regulate stress as much as possible. Let's pause and apply some Stress Away. (Pass your Stress Away around.) Now understand stress and the ECS is a two-way street. Although your endocannabinoid system helps balance your reaction to stress, chronic stress can lessen the ability of the ECS to do its job, which leaves you more vulnerable to the negative effects of stress.

We also need to take a premium probiotic supplement like Life-9. You probably already know that probiotics benefit digestive health, but they also support your ECS. Research is starting to show the beneficial effects of probiotic strains on the ECS. Life 9 has 17 billion live cultures from 9 beneficial bacteria strains. We need this bacteria to repopulate in our microbiome to maintain homeostasis.

For overall health, it is important to start making healthy lifestyle changes. What we feed our body matters. If we put in junk, we will feel like junk. Good nutrition is important for every system of the body. Sunshine and exercise are also a great way to support this lifestyle. The best source of vitamin D is Sunshine but if you can't always get out, a premium supplement, like Super Vitamin D, can help give your body a boost. Vitamin D deficiency is prevalent and has been linked to a number of autoimmune disorders, so get out outside and take your supplements. And yes, you guessed it, Vitamin D supplementation can also help to support CB2 receptor function.
We've talked a lot about the endocannabinoid system, diet, exercise and supplements, now let's talk about our CBD products that can tie all of this together.

NATURE'S ULTRA CBD

Smart Spectrum CBD is our own high-quality CBD isolate combined with essential oils from Young Living. It provides all of the benefits of pure, potent CBD infused with the best essential oils on earth. There's no other company in the world that uses this incredible formula.

Natures Ultra and Young Living partnered together to formulate their one of a kind Smart Spectrum CBD product. The hemp grown on our Young Living farm is organic and sustainable from beginning to end. They use a proprietary CO2 extraction to produce the highest quality CBD isolate you can get. Quality starts at the source; our farms and distilleries, then ends at your doorstep.

You can choose between one or all of our essential oil infused CBD drops such as cinnamon, citrus or cool mint. You can also get our unique CBD Beauty Oil, Calm Roll On, and CBD Muscle Rub. No matter which ones you choose, you are supporting your ECS.

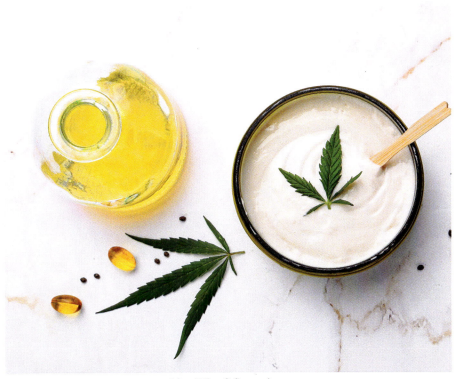

4-MONTH WELLNESS PLAN

The products we covered today are great examples of what you can put on your Subscribe to Save order to jump start your 4-Month Wellness Plan. But remember, everybody is different. Sometimes we have an immediate response using Young Living products. I am sure we all can agree that one drop of oil will not really support the underlying signals your body may be giving you. You need to make a commitment to use your products consistently. Be okay with that.

You've already started by being here. Now use your NOW WHAT? book to set up a 4-Month Wellness Plan. Check off the products you want to order each month on page xx.

Remember to personalize your choices. Look at the "You May Also Like" Products and choose from there, too. If you want to take it up a notch, you may want to incorporate the endocannabinoid raindrop products on page xx.

(Give the guests a few minutes to develop their plan. Be available to help them personalize, otherwise, sit back, be quiet and let them think.)

Okay, now that you all have your plan, pull out your smartphone and log onto your Shopping Platform. We are going to set up your first Subscribe to Save order. If you are not familiar with this yet, this will save you money while getting the products you need to get well. Remember, if you order more than 50pv you will earn free products through our Loyalty Rewards program too. All you have to do is make sure you consistently process 50pv every month to participate. I have your member number if you don't know it.

(Coach them through setting up their orders. You can send the guests a link to the My YL Bundle that corresponds with their health goal. Help them navigate the shopping platform and create their account.)

ENDOCANNABINOID SYSTEMS

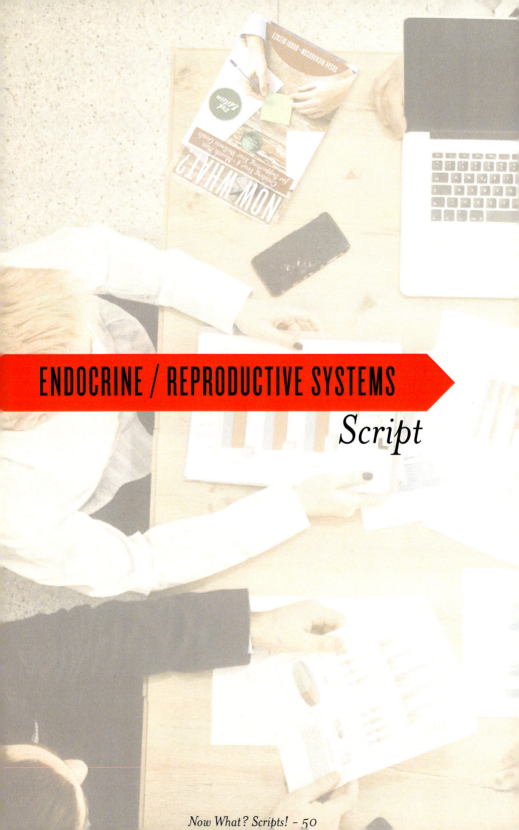

ENDOCRINE / REPRODUCTIVE SYSTEMS
Script

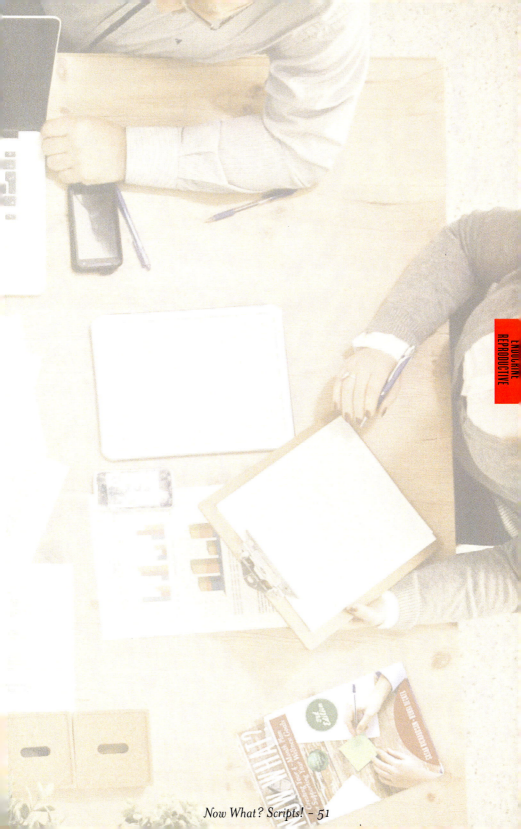

ENDOCRINE AND REPRODUCTIVE SYSTEMS
for both Men and Women

Hello everyone, in case you don't know me, my name is _____ . I am part of your Young Living Support Team. Thank you for being a part of our oily family. I want to thank (Host/Hostess) for opening up his/her home to us so we can learn more about how to take your health to the next level.

As Young Living customers, we all know what essential oils are and how they work in our bodies. Essential oils and essential oil-infused products are the number one way to protect your home from harsh chemicals and toxins; and promote health for you and your entire family.

Because Young Living is a health and wellness company, we are able to address wellness from a whole body perspective. And we can also look more in-depth at individual body systems like we are going to do today with the endocrine and reproductive systems.

This shouldn't shock you, but we discourage people from buying just a single oil. However, if that is what you choose, we recommend you put it on a Subscribe to Save order to help you save money. We don't want to mislead anyone into thinking one bottle of oil can help them achieve their health goals. Instead, we like to empower you with healthy lifestyle habits and to set up your own 4-Month Wellness Plan so you can reach and maintain your health goals.

With all of this in mind, let's take a closer look at the endocrine and reproductive systems. Open your Now What? book to the endocrine systems pages 12-15 or if your focus is on the reproductive system open to pages 26 and 27. The endocrine system has such a unique delivery system in that it sends hormones to targeted organs and tissues throughout the circulatory system. Having proper functioning endocrine and circulatory systems is vital in reproductive health. It is SO important to do everything you can to ensure you are getting the proper nutrition you need to support all of these mechanisms in your body. We know that when we use an essential oil-infused product it helps our

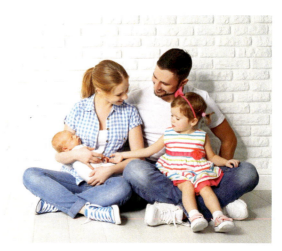

body absorb and distribute nutrition from the foods we eat and makes the nutrients from our supplements we take more bioavailable. We can even use the Vitality essential oils as dietary supplements.

There are also specific oils that have been shown to be incredibly supportive with certain gland and organ functions. Oils such as Lemon Vitality and Frankincense Vitality can be especially beneficial.

These Vitality essential oils can be easily added to your morning NingXia Red shot to support His and Her endocrine and reproductive systems. So let's all do a NingXia shot. **(Pass endocrine shots around.)**

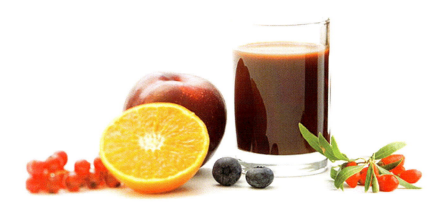

Frankincense Vitality is found in Cortistop™ for women and Prostate Health for men. Prostate Health is a unique formula for men to support the male glandular system and promote a healthy normal prostate function. The Coristop, likewise, is uniquely formulated to help women. How many women here experience stress? Pay attention! When you have stress, your body produces cortisol. If you are under stress frequently, too much cortisol can be produced causing negative health responses like fatigue, difficulty with weight management, and even difficulty maintaining cardiovascular health. Cortistop helps support the female glandular system and regulates normal cortisol production. Both of these products, Prostate Health and Cortistop, require consistent use to see optimum benefits.

Whether you are looking for healthy hormones, maintaining normal thyroid function, or looking for reproductive health, make sure you are putting good nutrients, a full range of amino acids, powerful B vitamins and protein in your diet. A simple solution: use our amazing Pure Protein Shake. This shake not only gives you good nutrition and 25 grams of protein, but will also enhance metabolism and Adenosine triphosphate or ATP production which is how your body produces energy.

NINGXIA RED

Could you use a little more energy? (Yes.)

Along with NingXia Red, Pure Protein Complete is an excellent whole food supplement that will enhance your diet and overall well-being, This makes NingXia Red and Pure Protein Complete a powerhouse for these systems.

What did you think of your NingXia Red shot? It was good, right? This is one way to kick start our morning; a happy endocrine system makes for a happy day. NingXia Red actually supports every system of the body. NingXia Red helps us to maintain that health, stamina, and cognitive wellness.

It is a funny name, but NingXia is actually the name of the province in China where the primary ingredient is grown. The NingXia wolfberry is the predominant food of the people in this region who live to be over 100 years old. They contribute their health and longevity to this particular wolfberry which is packed full of dense nutrition and contains 4x the nutrients of the wolfberries in neighboring provinces.

The endocrine system needs a diet rich in antioxidants, fiber, and healthy fats to work properly. NingXia Red is very high in antioxidants, which means that it helps support our body's natural defense against aging. Dr. Richard Cutler, National Institutes of Health said, "The amount of antioxidants that you maintain in your body is directly proportional to how long you live!"

There are actually 17 species of wolfberry but only the NingXia wolfberry has a complete phytonutrient profile. It is higher in vitamin C than oranges, higher in calcium than cauliflower and higher in betacarotene than carrots. It's also high in vitamin E which plays an important role in the health and the maintenance of a healthy reproductive system in women and men. Testes and ovaries both thrive on NingXia Red.

NingXia Red is also high in protein. It has amino acids which are important for healthy hormonal production and function and 21 trace minerals which are important for every system of the body to properly function. NingXia Red has six essential fatty acids which are important because our bodies don't produce essential fatty acids naturally; they must come from your diet. Essential fatty acids promote proper hormone production, thyroid function, and adrenal activity. Do you see how this all works together?

NingXia Red is loaded with naturally occurring B vitamins like B1, B2, and B6 and more. This is dense nutrition. And let's face it, most people are not getting what they need from the food they eat.

NingXia Red contains high quality juices and purees like blueberry, pomegranate, plum, and cherry. Amazingly, even with these juices included, it still supports healthy blood sugar levels. This is because it is a puree and contains the fruit fiber.

Another thing that sets NingXia Red apart is that it is the only nutritive supplement available that is infused with essential oils. This aids the body's ability to absorb and assimilate all of those nutrients offering whole body support including our emotional well-being.

Another excellent source of nutrition is Master Formula. While this product is listed under the men's 4-Month Wellness Plan, it is just as beneficial for women and is listed in the reproductive section as well. Master Formula is a supplement that provides core building blocks for the proper function of all body systems, including vitamins, probiotics, minerals, and omega-3 fatty acids.

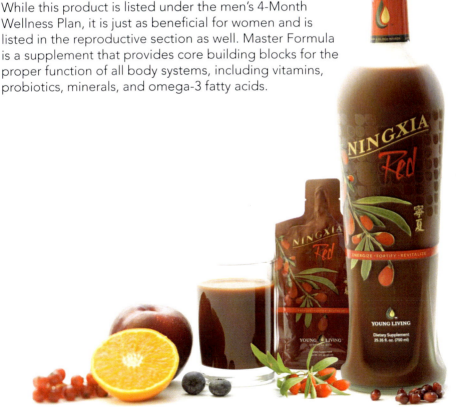

What is an endocrine/reproductive health class without talking about emotions?

If you're looking for a little calming or de-stressing, Clary Sage and Endoflex™ for women or Mister™ and Shutran™ for men should be your GO TOs for these systems. You can wear these topically on your ankles, big toes or wrists, or even just put it in your diffuser for a relaxing aroma, and these oils support self-esteem, confidence, hope, mental strength, libido and feelings of sexual desire for both women and men. Who knew?

Young Living also has a supplement called FemiGen™. This whole food supplement also contains herbs and amino acids. This is a perfect addition for women who are looking to balance and support the female reproductive system.

PowerGize was formulated to support the male reproductive system. It boosts stamina and performance, did you hear that? It contains herbs and essential oils that help sustain energy levels, enhances physical strength & endurance, and improves mental clarity.

You have heard us mention B vitamins several times. Super B is well known for its effect on positive moods, too. Young Living makes getting your Bs very easy with this comprehensive vitamin complex containing all eight essential, bioavailable energy-boosting B vitamins (B1, B2, B3, B5, B6, B7, B9, and B12). These Bs are in the best possible ratio to be absorbed by your body and contain folate, NOT folic acid, which is important for reproductive health.

Another great supplement for men and women is PD 80/20™. Once we hit the age of 20, naturally occurring DHEA and pregnenolone declines in men and women. Pregnenolone is known as the master hormone which is the precursor for estrogen, testosterone, and progesterone. This dietary supplement supports not only the endocrine system but also the immune and cardiovascular systems as well.

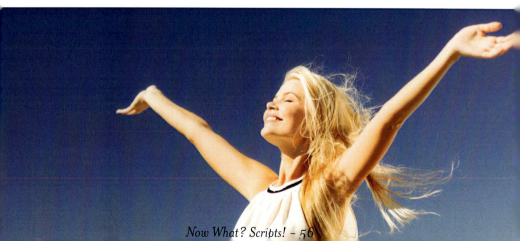

While it's important to provide your body with essential vitamins and nutrients that support your body systems, understand that it is equally as important to protect the outside of your body and your environment. Many times people will say they already use all natural personal care products. But what does that really mean? Did you know there are over 80,000 chemicals used in store-bought personal care products? Many of which have ingredients that legally don't have to be on the label? By using any of these, we create bioaccumulation and overload our systems with toxic chemicals and compromise our endocrine system.

What we put IN, ON, and AROUND our bodies matters!

Young Living has multiple product lines to increase your ability to stay healthy and transfer your personal care products from the box store products to Young Living's: Dragon Time™ Bath And Shower Gel and Mirah™ Shave Oil for women; and the Shutran 3™ in 1 Wash, Charcoal Bar Soap, Shutran Shave Cream and Aftershave Oil for men. And ladies, swap out your makeup with the Young Living's Savvy Minerals Makeup. Be sure to get the Orange Blossom Facial Wash & Moisturizer too. It will not only clean your face but nurture your skin. Your Endocrine System will thank you and you will looking smashing. Lastly, remember to replace your household cleaners with the Thieves clean living line.

Okay, ladies, listen up. There are two more essential oils blends we want to share. Progessence Plus™ is perfect for those of us over 30 years old. It contains wild yam and Vitamin E and can be nourishing to our skin. This is a perfect complementary product for your endocrine and reproductive 4-Month Wellness Plan. If you are moving past 50, Transformation™ would be a perfect choice for you. This is especially for women who have negative self-talk about this new stage of life. This powerful blend will empower you through with uplifting thoughts.

4-MONTH WELLNESS PLAN

The products we covered today are great examples of what you can put on your Subscribe to Save order to jump start your 4-Month Wellness Plan. But remember, everybody is different. Sometimes we have an immediate response using Young Living products, but I am sure we all can agree that one drop of oil will not really support the underlying signals your body may be giving you. You need to make a commitment to use your products consistently. Be okay with that.

You've already started by being here. Now use your NOW WHAT? book to set up a 4-Month Wellness Plan. Check off the products you want to order each month on page 13 or 15.

AND REMEMBER… when personalizing your choices, look at the "You May Also Like" Products on the previous pages too.

(Give the guests a few minutes to develop their plan. Be available to help them personalize, otherwise, sit back, be quiet and let them think.)

Okay, now that you all have your plan, pull out your smartphone and log onto your Shopping Platform. We are going to set up your first month's order with Subscribe to Save. If you are not familiar with this yet, this will save you money while getting the products you need to get well. Remember, if you order more than 50pv you will earn free products through our Loyalty Rewards program too. All you have to do is make sure you consistently process 50pv every month to participate. I have your member number if you don't know it.

(Coach them through setting up their order. You can send the guests a link to the My YL Bundle that corresponds with their health goal. Help them navigate the shopping platform and create their account.)

ENDOCRINE REPRODUCTIVE

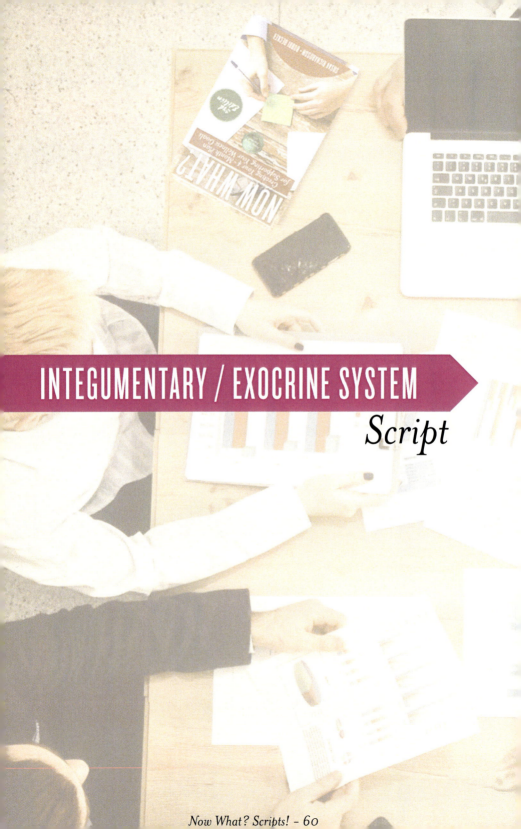

INTEGUMENTARY / EXOCRINE SYSTEM
Script

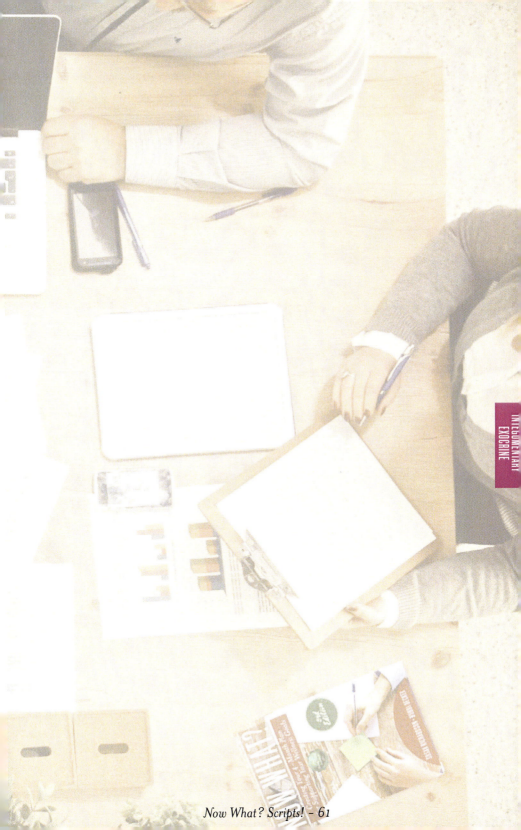

Hello everyone, in case you don't know me, my name is _____ . I am part of your Young Living Support Team. Thank you for being a part of our oily family. I want to thank (Host/Hostess) for opening up his/her home to us so we can learn more about how to take your health to the next level.

As Young Living customers, we all know what essential oils are and how they work in our bodies. Essential oils and essential oil-infused products are the number one way to protect your home from harsh chemicals and toxins; and promote health for you and your entire family.

Because Young Living is a health and wellness company, we are able to address wellness from a whole body perspective. And we can also look more in-depth at individual body systems like we are going to do today with the integumentary system.

This shouldn't shock you, but we discourage people from buying just a single oil. However, if that is what you choose, we recommend you put it on a Subscribe to Save oder to help you save money. We don't want to mislead anyone into thinking one bottle of oil can help them achieve their health goals. Instead, we like to empower you with healthy lifestyle habits and to set up your own 4-Month Wellness Plan so you can reach and maintain your health goals.

With all this in mind, let's take a closer look at the integumentary system.

So open your Now What? book to the Integumentary System on pages 16 and 17.

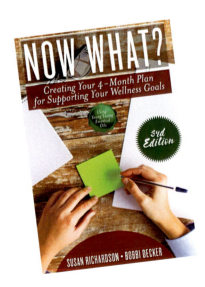

This system of our body works like essential oils do for our plants in that it protects our body from environmental stressors. It contains connective tissues, vessels, glands, follicles, hair roots, nails, sensory nerve endings, and muscular tissue. The skin is the largest organ in the body. This system is our first line of defense, so let's make sure we take care of it.

We know that when we use an essential oil-infused product, it helps our body absorb and distribute nutrition from the foods we eat and makes the nutrients from our supplements we take more bioavailable. This is one reason we use the Vitality essential oils as dietary supplements. So looking at this list of Vitality Oils, you should already have some of these Vitality oils like Lemon, and the classic oils like Lavender and Frankincense.

Young Living also has Carrot Seed and Rosemary Vitality which are well known for supporting skin and hair health. You can easily add any of these or any combination of them to your morning NingXia Red shot to support your integumentary system every morning. In fact, let's try a NingXia Red shot now. (Pass integumentary shots around.)

NingXia Red is the supplement everyone should be drinking daily. We recommend that this be the first thing you put on your 4-Month Wellness Plan, regardless of the system you are supporting.

This is because NingXia Red supports every system of the body. Even for those of us who are already healthy, NingXia Red helps us to maintain that health, stamina, and cognitive wellness.

It is a funny name, but NingXia is actually the name of the province in China where the primary ingredient is grown. The NingXia wolfberry is the predominant food of the people in this region who live to be over 100 years old. They contribute their health and longevity to this particular wolfberry which is packed full of dense nutrition and contains 4x the nutrients of the wolfberries in neighboring provinces.

Antioxidants are really important for your hair, skin and entire integumentary system. NingXia Red is very high in antioxidants, which means that it helps support our body's natural defense against aging and neutralizes free radicals. Dr. Richard Cutler, National Institutes of Health said, "The amount of antioxidants that you maintain in your body is directly proportional to how long you live!" (See page 36-37 in Now What? for more antioxidant options).

There are actually 17 species of wolfberry but only the NingXia wolfberry has a complete phytonutrient profile. It is higher in vitamin C than oranges. Vitamin C is important in the role of the production of collagen to enhance a more youthful appearance.

NingXia wolfberries are also higher in calcium than cauliflower. And the wolfberries are higher in betacarotene than carrots. The body converts beta-carotene into vitamin A; we need vitamin A for healthy skin. It's also high in vitamin E which blocks free radicals from the body. This can help your skin look more youthful, too.

Your hair, skin, and nails are mostly made up of protein. NingXia Red is also high in protein which will help you maintain them. NingXia Red has amino acids which are important for healthy skin and collagen, as well as other body functions. It has 21 trace minerals which are important for all of the systems of the body to properly function, 6 essential fatty acids, vitamins B1, B2, and B6 and more. This is dense nutrition not just for our skin and integumentary system, but for the whole body.

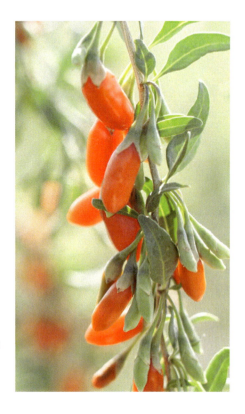

It contains high quality juices and purees like blueberry, pomegranate, plum, and cherry. Amazingly, even with these juices included, it still supports healthy blood sugar levels. This is because it is a puree and contains the fruit fiber.

NingXia Red is the foundation for every system, so it stands to reason that it is the first addition to your 4-Month Wellness Plan. It doesn't matter what your goal is, this is our #1 choice for everyone.

As we know, all health begins in the digestive system. And the health of your integumentary system is directly linked to the health of your gut. So, along with NingXia Red, Life 9 is a great supplement to use. Life 9 is pretty amazing because it has 9 clinically proven high-potency probiotic strains that work well together. It combines 17 billion live cultures from these 9 bacteria strains that promote healthy digestion, supports gut health, and helps maintain normal intestinal function for overall health.

Enzymes make digestion and absorption of nutrients possible. This is why NingXia Red, Life 9, and enzymes work together. Essentialzyme enhances enzyme activity and supports the pancreas while Detoxzyme supports detoxification and cleansing, while supporting overall health. Both are necessary for a healthy system.

Consuming prebiotics is important to these mechanisms as well. Prebiotics feed the good microbes in the gut. You can easily obtain these by adding ICP Daily or Sulfurzyme Powder to your NingXia Red. Not only does this taste amazing, but every mechanism of our body and every cell needs sulfur (MSM) to function, so it is an important addition to our healthy regimen. The MSM is formulated with the NingXia wolfberry which contains minerals and coenzymes that the sulfur needs to assimilate and metabolize. Sulfurzyme supports the integumentary system and promotes clear skin. Sulfur is vital in maintaining the structure of proteins, protects cellular function and cell membranes, and supports connective tissue. And keeping with the seed to seal promise, Young Living sources their MSM from sources that we can trust and it tests every single batch for mercury, lead, pesticides, and more to ensure it's purity.

When we take care of our microbiome, benefits are vast. It will give us the ability to stay active, sustain energy, and promote nutrient absorption (such as folate). Young Living makes getting your B's very easy with Super B, a comprehensive vitamin complex containing all eight essential, bioavailable energy-boosting B vitamins (B1, B2, B3, B5, B6, B7, B9, and B12). These B's are in the best possible ratio to be absorbed by your body and contains folate, NOT folic acid, which is vital for skin and hair health.

What is an integumentary class without talking about personal care products like shampoo, facial wash, and skin nourishment?

What we put IN, ON and AROUND our bodies matters!

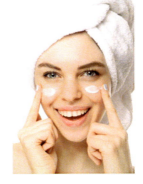

While it's important to provide your body with essential vitamins and nutrients that support your body systems, understand that it is as equally important to protect the outside of your body and your environment. Many times people will say they already use all natural personal care products.

Now What? Scripts! - 65

But what does that really mean? Did you know there are over 80,000 chemicals used in store-bought personal care products? Women, alone, are exposed to well over 300 chemicals before they even sit down for breakfast. Many personal care products have ingredients that legally don't have to be listed on the label. By using any of these, we create bio-accumulation and overload our systems with harsh chemicals and compromise our health.

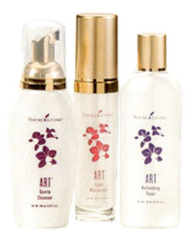

Young Living has many safe products to increase your ability to nourish your hair and skin. Remember when you are in a hot shower, your pores open up, so what you are shampooing with will absorb into your body when it runs down your body. You can be rest assured that all of Young Living's shampoos and conditioners are plant derived, safe and formulated to leave your hair healthy and clean. There also may be an adjustment time with the personal care products as we switch from harsh products to plant-based ingredients. Young Living products are super concentrated, so less is more.

There are a variety of skin care products that you can choose from depending on your skin needs. You can look through pages 32-35 of your Now What? book or simply go with the Orange Blossom Facial Wash which contains MSM and Lavender essential oil to soften and support sensitive skin. This is a very gentle soap-free cleanser which helps remove impurities without stripping away your natural balance of oils. Then choose a moisturizer like the Orange Blossom Moisturizer or the ART light moisturizer.

A few more skin care products that would be perfect to add to your 4-Month Wellness Plan would be LavaDerm, Mirah Shave Oil, and Cel-Lite. Cel-Lite tones and nourishes the skin with pure vegetable oils, vitamin E, and essential oils like Grapefruit to improve the appearance of the skin's texture and Juniper to help with cleansing. LavaDerm Cooling Mist contains Lavender, Helichrysum, aloe and ionic trace minerals to soothe and rejuvenate skin when overexposed to the elements.

Plus, we have an amazing Savvy Minerals Makeup Line. This makeup will nourish and protect your skin without fillers, synthetics, or parabens, and as a perfect complement to these products you can use the Mirah Cleansing Oil and other Mirah products. The Cleansing oil is gentle and safe and works great as a makeup remover. Mirrah is formulated with ten essential oils, including Rose and Ylang Ylang, and contains ten moisturizing carrier oils, like jojoba and argan, this facial cleanser removes pore-clogging impurities without stripping away the natural oils your skin needs. There are many other options because we know that everyone's skin is different.

4-MONTH WELLNESS PLAN

The products we covered today are great examples of what you can put on your Subscribe to Save order to jump start your 4-Month Wellness Plan. But remember, everybody's skin and hair care needs are different. Look through the Anti-Aging section starting on page 30 and through the "You May Also Like" products listed on page 14 to determine your own personalized wellness plan.

If you are personalizing for a child, you may want to incorporate the KidScents™ products on page 43.

Instruct your customers to review the products and set up their 4-Month Wellness Plan.

(Give the guests a few minutes to develop their plan. Be available to help them personalize, otherwise, sit back, be quiet and let them think.)

Okay, now that you all have your plan, pull out your smartphone and log into your virtual office. We are going to set up your Subscribe to Save order. If you are not familiar with this yet, this will save you money while getting the products you need to get well. Remember, if you order more than 50pv you will earn free products through our Loyalty Rewards program too. All you have to do is make sure you consistently process 50pv every month to participate. I have your member number if you don't know it.

(Coach them through setting up their order. You can send the guests a link to the My YL Bundle that corresponds with their health goal. Help them navigate the shopping platform and create their account.)

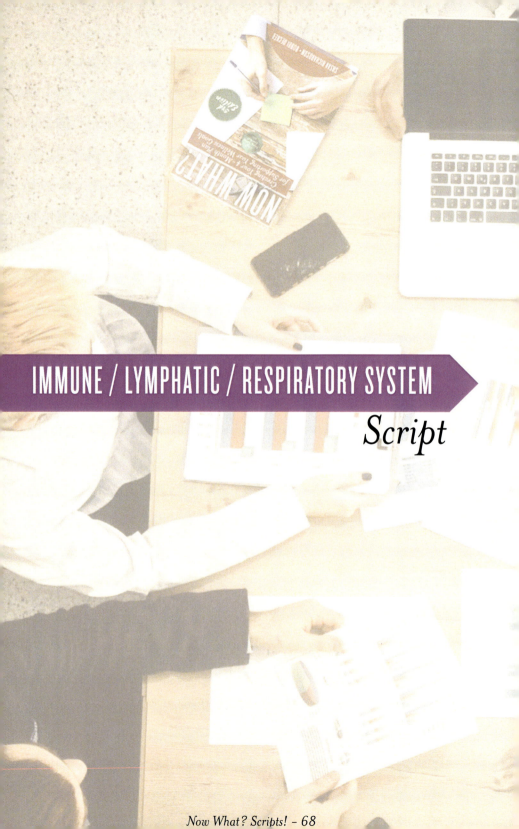

IMMUNE / LYMPHATIC / RESPIRATORY SYSTEM Script

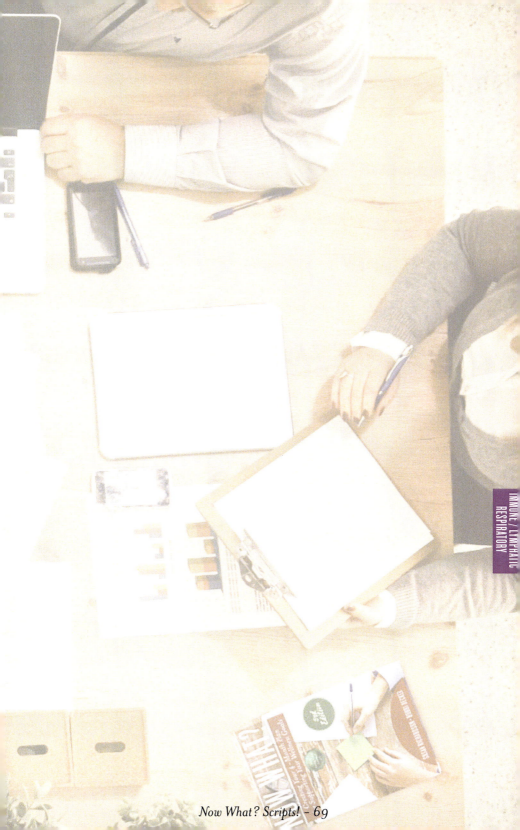

IMMUNE / LYMPHATIC / RESPIRATORY

Hello everyone, in case you don't know me, my name is _____ . I am your part of your Young Living Support Team. Thank you for being a part of our oily family. I want to thank (Host/Hostess) for opening up his/her home to us so we can learn more about how to take your health to the next level.

As Young Living customers, we all know what essential oils are and how they work in our bodies. Essential oils and essential oil-infused products are the number one way to protect your home from harsh chemicals and toxins; and promote health for you and your entire family.

Because Young Living is a health and wellness company, we are able to address wellness from a whole body perspective. And we can also look more in-depth at individual body systems like we are going to do today with the immune and respiratory systems.

This shouldn't shock you, but we discourage people from buying just a single oil. However, if that is what you choose, we recommend you put it on a Subscribe to Save oder to help you save money. We don't want to mislead anyone into thinking one bottle of oil can help them achieve their health goals. Instead, we like to empower you with healthy lifestyle habits and to set up your own 4-Month Wellness Plan so you can reach and maintain your health goals.

With all this in mind, let's take a close look at the immune and respiratory systems and discuss a few ways to address these systems of the body so that you can keep them above the health line.

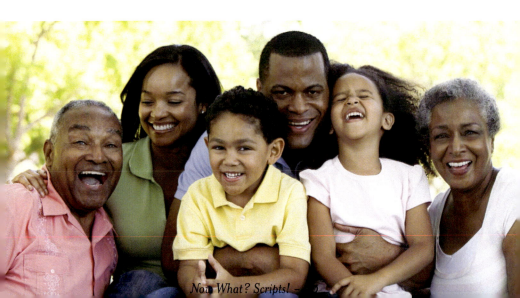

For most people, stress is a normal part of life and comes from a range of places such as school, your job or even your family. It doesn't matter if it's good stress that acts as a motivator to help you "get the job done" or cumulative stress from taking care of a loved one. Stress is Stress. Dr. Leonard Calabrese says, "Eliminating or modifying stress factors in life is vital to protect and augment the immune response and is necessary to buffer the inevitability of the aging process." So, YES, stress affects both immune function and aging.

Stress happens when life events surpass your ability to cope and causes the stress hormone cortisol to flood your body. Cortisol is a great thing in moderation and can boost your immune system. But too much cortisol will increase inflammation and lower immune function which puts musculoskeletal system at risk for tense muscles, respiratory function distress, and even depression and anxiety from an imbalanced nervous system.

An overly tired immune system loses its ability to protect you, so what can you do to help your body stay more relaxed and calm? Breathe, just take in a few deep breaths. Deep breathing helps boost your immune system and stimulates your lymphatic system to filter out toxins and relaxes you. Meditating 10 to 15 minutes a day has been clinically proven to lower stress levels and reduce cortisol levels and reduce inflammation - or you can do a little yoga.

Let's take 20 seconds to oxygenate our bodies… Close your eyes and take in 3 deep cleansing breaths.

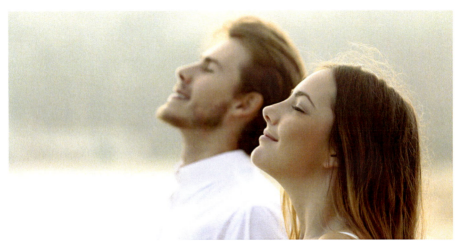

Now that we are calm and relaxed, open your Now What? book to the immune system on page 18 (or page 28, if you are here to focus on the respiratory system). The immune system is a network of lymphatic vessels which defends the body against disease, fights infection, recycles plasma proteins, and drains the fluid back into the circulatory system. This helps you stay hydrated and above the health line.

The respiratory system carries oxygen-rich air to your lungs and carbon dioxide and waste gas out of your lungs. This includes your nose and linked air passages, mouth, larynx, trachea, and bronchial tubes.

These two systems work hand-in-hand with the digestive system, so we need to ensure that we are getting the proper nutrition we need to support every system of the body. We know that when we use an essential oil-infused product, it helps our body absorb and distribute nutrition from the foods we eat and makes the nutrients from the supplements we take more bioavailable. You should already have some Vitality oils and Classic Essential Oils. Whatever you have, make sure you pull them out and use them every day. We recommend you get Thieves, DiGize and Lemon Vitality, if you don't already have them; and add Frankincense and Lavender to your collection too.

You can easily add the Vitality Oils to your morning NingXia Red shot to support your Immune System every morning. So let's all do a NingXia shot while we discuss NingXia Red. (Pass Immune NingXia Red shots around.)

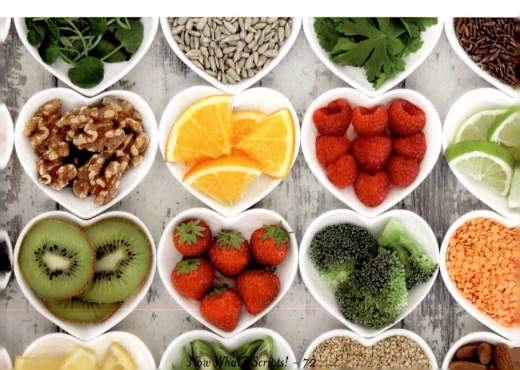

NingXia Red supports every system of the body, even for those of us who are already healthy. NingXia Red helps us to maintain that health, stamina, and cognitive wellness. But today we are going to focus on supporting respiratory and immune health.

NingXia Red is the supplement everyone should be drinking daily. We recommend that this be the first thing you put on your 4-Month Wellness Plan, regardless of the system you are supporting.

It is a funny name, but NingXia is actually the name of the province in China where the primary ingredient is grown. The NingXia wolfberry is the predominant food of the people in this region who live to be over 100 years old. They contribute their health and longevity to this particular wolfberry which is packed full of dense nutrition and contains 4x the nutrients of the wolfberries in neighboring provinces.

NingXia Red is very high in antioxidants, which means that it helps support our body's natural defense against aging. Dr. Richard Cutler, National Institutes of Health said, "The amount of antioxidants that you maintain in your body is directly proportional to how long you live!" Antioxidants are also important to immune function; free radicals damage your immune cells and inhibit communication between cells. Fueling your body with antioxidants is going to protect and fortify your immune system.

There are actually 17 species of wolfberry and only the Ningxia wolfberry has a complete phytonutrient profile. These wolfberries are higher in vitamin C than oranges. Vitamin C's role in boosting the immune system is well researched. Studies show it increases the production of white blood cells, antibodies, and stimulates the cell to heighten its natural defenses. (Research interferon!) Do you want an extra Vitamin C boost? Young Living's Super C has 1440% of the RDA (recommended daily allowance) per serving and a proprietary blend to ensure bioavailability. Together, Super C and NingXia are a powerhouse for the immune system.

Another thing that sets NingXia Red apart is that it is the only nutritive supplement available that is infused with essential oils. This aids the body's ability to absorb and assimilate all of those nutrients offering whole body support on a cellular level.

MultiGreens is another whole food supplement that is designed to work with not only our lymphatic and immune system, but respiratory system, too. MultiGreens contains a natural algae, spirulina, that is high in antioxidants, B vitamins and other nutrients that fill in the gaps of our diets. This live green food contains other immune stimulating ingredients like bee pollen and choline.

Another supplement that you can use regularly to enhance immune and respiratory system health is Inner Defense. Inner Defense is basically Thieves Vitality in a capsule combined with the proper ratio of Thyme Vitality, Oregano Vitality and Lemongrass Vitality for extra support. Inner Defense creates an unfriendly terrain for yeast and fungus in your gut. It tends to be most effective when taken 6-8 hours before our probiotic, Life 9. Life 9 is pretty amazing because it has 9 clinically proven high-potency probiotic strains that do not inhibit each other. It combines 17 billion live cultures from these 9 bacteria strains that promote healthy digestion, gut health, and helps maintain normal intestinal function. These two products together are a powerhouse for your immune system.

Young Living has multiple product lines to increase your ability to stay healthy. Replace the harsh chemicals in your home with the Thieves products. This clean living line includes the household cleaner, hand soap, toothpaste, mouthwash, hand sanitizer and even a misting spray to conveniently use when you are out and about (you can use that on door knobs, shopping carts or even toilets). The thieves products are going to replace all of your cleaning supplies and many of your personal care items that impede your immune system and health.

This product line is 100% natural and safe so you can feel good about using it around your family and pets. We can use this household cleaner on everything from lunch boxes to toilets. This plant based formula uses a naturally occurring surfactant derived from coconut and is non abrasive, leaves behind no chemical residue and is safe for septic systems. It is highly concentrated, making it cost effective! *(Hold up pre-diluted spray bottle.)* This bottle is my all purpose cleaner. I add one cap of the Thieves Household Cleaner and fill the rest with water. I use this on everything.

By using these products, you will protect your home from harsh chemicals that can compromise your health while saving you money. And, it doesn't matter if you are brushing your teeth or scrubbing your toilet, you are supporting your immune and respiratory health when you use any of the Thieves products.

Thieves Vitality supports a healthy immune and respiratory system and protects our body's natural defenses. We can take this as a supplement in a gel cap or we can add it to a warm cup of water and honey. We use the classic blend to diffuse and purify our air or we rub it on the bottoms of our feet.

The NON-Young Living personal care products that we are buying in box stores such as laundry detergent, lotions, shampoos, bath and body products and even oils are made with toxic chemicals and fragrances. These are made in factories and laboratories, not grown in a field. The harsh chemicals from these other products compromise not only our immune and respiratory systems, but every system of the body.

It is super easy to integrate them into your daily lifestyle by ordering them through Young Living's Subscribe to Save program. Just select the products you want, the frequency you want them, and have them shipped to your front door.

Did you know that store-bought laundry detergent has optical brighteners added? These brighteners give the illusion of our clothes being clean and bright. The frightening fact is that these chemicals used to give this appearance don't just stay on and in your clothing, but when you smell those fragrances, those same chemicals are being spread throughout your body through you skin, lungs, and respiratory system.

In the same way, every time we wash our dishes, we are absorbing chemicals like sodium lauryl sulfate which can be in a ratio as high as 30%. This level is considered unsafe and is affecting your respiratory and immune systems. This is not just in your dish soap but is also found in toothpaste, mouthwash, makeup, body wash and shampoos. Sodium lauryl sulfate (SLS) is known to be a "moderate hazard" and has been linked to cancer, neurotoxicity, organ toxicity, skin irritation and endocrine disruption and yet it is one of the most commonly used ingredients in shampoos.

And did you know your mouth tissue absorbs even more? When you put a substance in your mouth, it is absorbed more quickly and thoroughly. Anything going under the tongue bypasses the entire digestive system and delivers it straight to the bloodstream. No waiting, no roadblocks — just straight into the blood. So when we use store-bought toothpaste or mouthwash, we are putting these chemicals right into our bloodstream. Think about that!

Wouldn't it be great to be able to clean your house, wash your dishes, and even brush your teeth without compromising your health?

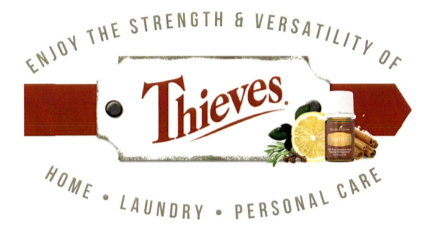

4 MONTH WELLNESS PLAN

The products we covered today are great examples of what you can put on your Subscribe to Save order to jump start your 4-Month Wellness Plan. Remember, everybody is different, sometimes we have an immediate response using Young Living products, but I am sure we all can agree that one drop of oil will not really support the underlying signals your body may be giving you. You need to make a commitment to use your products consistently. Be okay with that.

You've already started by being here. Now use your NOW WHAT? book to set up a 4-Month Wellness Plan. Check off the products you want to order each month on page 19 and/or page 29.

And remember to personalize your choices. Look at the "You May Also Like" Products and choose from there, too. If you are personalizing for a child, you may want to incorporate the KidScents products found on page 43. If you want to take it up a notch, you may want to incorporate the Raindrop products.

(Give the guests a few minutes to develop their plan. Be available to help them personalize, otherwise, sit back, be quiet and let them think.)

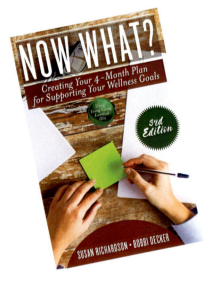

Okay, now that you all have your plan, pull out your smartphone and log onto your Shopping Platform. We are going to set up your first Subscribe to Save order.

If you are not familiar with this yet, this will save you money while getting the products you need to get well. Remember, if you order more than 50pv you will earn free products through our Loyalty Rewards program too. All you have to do is make sure you consistently process 50pv every month to participate. I have your member number if you don't know it.

(Coach them through setting up their order. You can send the guests a link to the My YL Bundle that corresponds with their health goal. Help them navigate the shopping platform and create their account.)

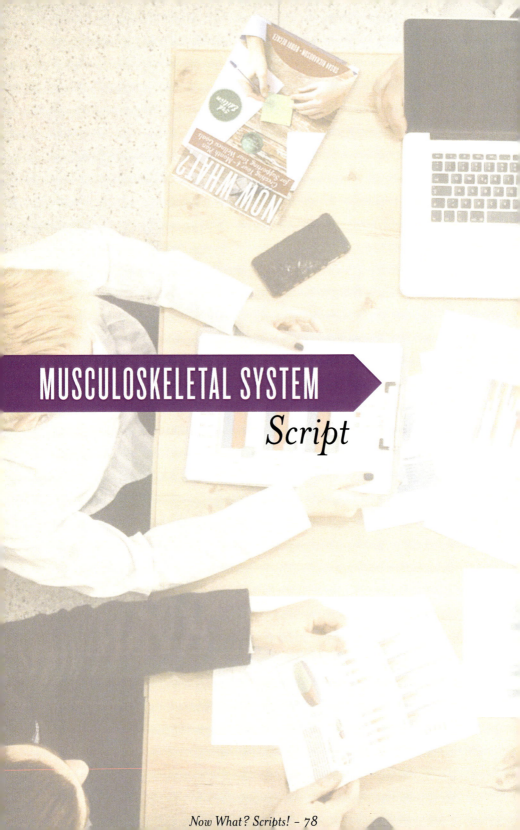

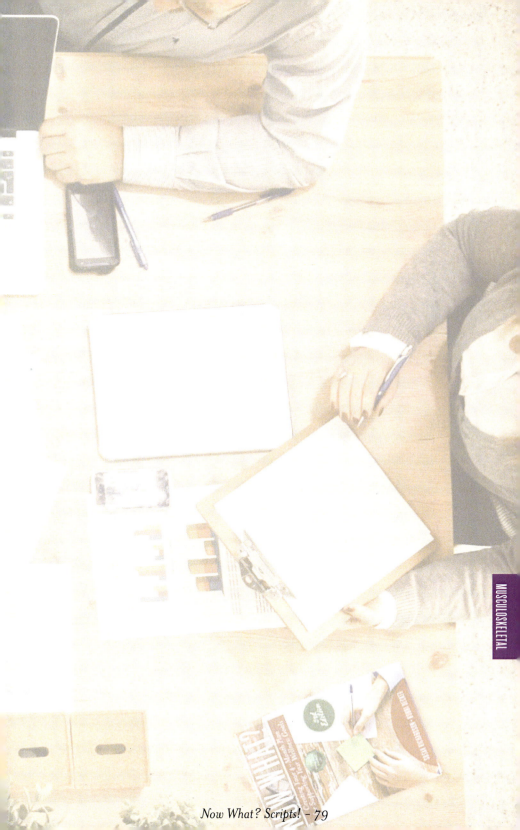

MUSCULOSKELETAL SYSTEM

Hello everyone, in case you don't know me, my name is _____ . I am a part of your Young Living Support Team. Thank you for being a part of our oily family. I want to thank (Host/Hostess) for opening up his/her home to us so we can learn more about how to take your health to the next level.

As Young Living customers, we all know what essential oils are and how they work in our bodies. Essential oils and essential oil-infused products are the number one way to protect your home from harsh chemicals and toxins; and promote health for you and your entire family.

Because Young Living is a health and wellness company, we are able to address wellness from a whole body perspective. And we can also look more in-depth at individual body systems like we are going to do today with the musculoskeletal system.

This shouldn't shock you, but we discourage people from buying just a single oil. However, if that is what you choose, we recommend you put it on a Subscribe to Save oder to help you save money. We don't want to mislead anyone into thinking one bottle of oil can help them achieve their health goals. Instead, we like to empower you with healthy lifestyle habits and to set up your own 4-Month Wellness Plan so you can reach and maintain your health goals.

With all this in mind, let's take a close look at the musculoskeletal system and discuss a few ways to address this system of the body so you can keep it above the health line.

So, open your Now What? book to the Musculoskeletal System on page 20 and 21. This system enables the body to move. It also supports your body and its organs, bones, joints, and ligaments.

It is SO important to do everything you can to ensure you and your family are getting the proper nutrition you need to support every system of your body.

We know that when we use an essential oil-infused product, it helps our body absorb and distribute nutrition from the foods we eat and makes the nutrients from the supplements we take more bioavailable. We can even use the Vitality essential oils as dietary supplements. You should already have some Vitality oils and Classic Essential Oils. Whatever you have, make sure you pull them out and use them every day. We recommend you get Peppermint and Frankincense Vitality, if you don't already have them.

Lemongrass Vitality is well known for supporting your bones, ligaments, and muscles, relieves body aches, and supports your body's natural response to inflammation. You can easily add a drop of Lemongrass and Copaiba Vitality to your morning NingXia Red shot to support your musculoskeletal system.

So let's all do a NingXia shot while we discuss NingXia Red. (Pass musculoskeletal shots around.)

NingXia Red is the supplement everyone should be drinking daily. We recommend that this be the first thing you put on your 4-Month Wellness Plan regardless of the system you are supporting.

It is a funny name, but NingXia is actually the name of the province in China where the primary ingredient is grown. The NingXia wolfberry is the predominant food of the people in this region who live to be over 100 years old. They contribute their health and longevity to this particular wolfberry which is packed full of dense nutrition and contains 4x the nutrients of the wolfberries in neighboring provinces.

NingXia Red is very high in antioxidants, and because of its high antioxidant level, has proven to help with the body's natural response to inflammation and helps support our body's natural defense against aging. Dr. Richard Cutler of the National Institutes of Health said, "The amount of antioxidants that you maintain in your body is directly proportional to how long you live!"

There are actually 17 species of wolfberry but only the NingXia Wolfberry has a complete phytonutrient profile. It is higher in vitamin C than oranges. Vitamin C's role in supporting bone health is well researched. Studies show it enhances the body's ability to strengthen bone density and strength. Do you want an extra Vitamin C boost? Young Living's Super C has 1440% the RDA (recommended daily allowance) per serving and a proprietary blend to ensure bioavailability. Together, Super C and NingXia Red are a powerhouse.

NingXia Red is also higher in calcium than cauliflower. Your body cannot create calcium so you need to get it from the foods you eat. And if your body doesn't absorb enough from the foods you eat, you must supplement it with quality nutrition like NingXia Red. Calcium is very important for the musculoskeletal system by helping your muscles, bones, and nerves work properly.

NingXia Red is also high in other nutrients like beta-carotene, vitamin E, and protein. It has amino acids which are important for musculoskeletal health and repair. Amino acids promote collagen, cartilage, and tendon formation. AminoWise would be the perfect complementary supplement to add to NingXia Red. (You could teach an entire class on AminoWise and BCAA's... do your research).

NingXia Red contains 21 trace minerals which are important for all of the systems of the body to properly function, 6 essential fatty acids, vitamins B1, B2, and B6 and more. This is dense nutrition. And let's face it, most people are not getting what they need from the food they eat.

It contains high quality juices and purees like blueberry, pomegranate, plum, and cherry. Amazingly, even with these juices included, it still supports healthy blood sugar levels. This is because it is a puree and contains the fruit fiber.

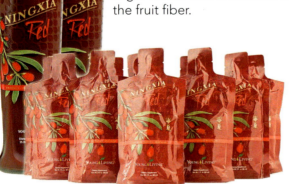

Another thing that sets NingXia Red apart is that it is the only nutritive supplement available that is infused with essential oils. This aids the body's ability to absorb and assimilate all of those nutrients offering whole body support including our emotional well-being.

AgilEase is formulated for individuals who want active lifestyles. With unique and powerful ingredients such as Frankincense powder, undenatured collagen, hyaluronic acid, and calcium fructoborate this supplement supports joint health. This supplement is especially beneficial for athletes, middle-aged, and elderly people who may experience a natural, acute joint discomfort and supports the body's natural response to acute inflammation. AgilEase is perfect for healthy individuals who are looking to gain greater mobility and flexibility.

Let's talk a little bit about physical activity because while diet and nutrition are important, it's good to move your body. The American Heart Association recommends for a healthy heart you must get 150 minutes of moderate exercise a week. Being physically active is important in preventing osteoporosis. Just 30 minutes of walking a day will decrease your chances of falling below the health line. So let's all stand up and move. Change seats and sit by someone new. Seriously, let's get up and move.

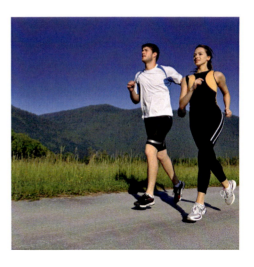

AgilEase is infused with essential oils like Wintergreen, Clove, and Copaiba. Copaiba Vitality is a powerful essential oil from Brazil that has been traditionally used to support the body's natural response to injury and inflammation. AgilEase and Copaiba Vitality are an amazing combination when used together to help support your body's musculoskeletal system.

Young Living is the only essential oil company that has registered over the counter (OTC) medication. This is a big deal. Young Living has worked closely with the FDA to get OTCs like the Cool Azul Pain Cream. This product combines Wintergreen and Peppermint essential oils to specifically address the musculoskeletal system. This pain cream provides relief from minor muscle and joint aches to arthritis, strains, bruises, and sprains. The active ingredient Methyl salicylate (methyl sal-i-cy-late) found in Wintergreen helps alleviate pain deep in the muscles and joints and the natural menthol found in Peppermint provides a cooling effect.

Does anyone here have pain? (Pass the pain cream around. Let them put a little on. If you have the CBD Joint and Muscle Rub instead, offer them this. Use a toothpick to distribute.)

AminoWise is a supplement that provides branched chain amino acids. The BCAs support muscles during AND after exercise to fight fatigue and enhance recovery. More than just an amino acid supplement, it's triple-targeted with branded chain amino acid for muscle building and repair, polyphenol and antioxidants for recovery, and a hydrating mineral blend to replace important minerals lost during exercise. AminoWise reduces lactic acid, enhances and recovery while decreasing recovery time.

Paired with a healthy diet, BCAs help create lean muscle mass AND muscle repair. The lemon-wolfberry flavored powder is added to water or NingXia Red. It contains no artificial colors or sweeteners, no sugar, and no dyes!!!

Okay, let's talk about PowerGize™. This supplement contains some exotic herbs and essential oils that support stamina, mental and physical vitality, performance and strength. It can help you maintain balanced energy and performance levels as well as support the entire musculoskeletal system.

Our supplements undergo the same meticulous process and standards as our essential oils. The fish oil in our OmegaGize3 exceeds purity standards and is sustainable. The sourced omega-3 in this product is one of the purest fish oils available and is rigorously and independently tested to ensure that it is free of environmental pollutants.

OmegaGize3 combines the power of three core daily supplements: omega-3 fatty acids, vitamin D3, and CoQ10. Vitamin D3 is a fat-soluble vitamin that may help improve the body's ability to absorb calcium in the gut. AND as we know, all health begins in the digestive system, even our musculoskeletal system.

4-MONTH WELLNESS PLAN

We have discussed NingXia Red and that it is the foundation for every system so it stands to reason that it is the first addition to your 4-Month Wellness Plan. It doesn't matter what your goal is, this is our #1 choice for everyone.

Let's also talk about MindWise. This is an AMAZING supplement that everyone should be taking along with their NingXia Red. The MindWise proprietary memory blend features ALCAR (acetyl-L-carnitine). *This functions as an antioxidant and promotes the production of glutathione and is a free radical scavenger. Research shows that glutathione supplementation improves lipid metabolism and acidification in skeletal muscles during exercise, leading to less muscle fatigue.*

MindWise also has glycerophosphocholine or GPC, a natural physiological precursor to a neurotransmitter that is involved in memory and other cognitive functions and is known to cross the blood brain barrier. Clinical studies have demonstrated it helps to support cognitive function and mental acuity as well as the development of lean muscle mass. Deficiencies in GPC can lead to problems with the musculoskeletal system.

CoQ10 is found in every cell of the body and is necessary for the basic functioning of cells and has been studied for supporting healthy brain function. CoQ10 supplementation has also been documented to show sustained cholesterol levels, circulatory function and normal overall heart and cardiovascular health. BUT NOT ONLY THAT… The National Library of Medicine and the National Institutes of Health report that supplementation of CoQ10 will improve anaerobic and/or aerobic exercise performance.

MindWise also contains Medium Chain Triglycerides *(MCT) from coconut oil and generous amounts of vitamin D3, both promoting musculoskeletal health. MCTs increase thermogenesis which means more calories burned and higher total energy expenditure. They increase fat oxidation, and increase the thermic effect of your food. They even may help preserve muscle mass. They are a fast acting energy source and are often marketed to athletes. Research from Johns Hopkins University found that people fed MCTs ate 87-102 calories less at the next meal.*

The products we covered today are great examples of what you can put on your Subscribe to Save order to jump start your 4-Month Wellness Plan. But remember, everybody is different, and sometimes we have an immediate response using Young Living products. I am sure we all can agree that one drop of oil will not really support the underlying signals your body may be giving you. You need to make a commitment to use your products consistently. Be okay with that.

You've already started by being here. Now use your NOW WHAT? book to set up a 4-Month Wellness Plan. Check off the products you want to order each month on page 21.

And remember to personalize your choices. Look at the "You May Also Like" Products and choose from there, too. If you are personalizing for a child, you may want to incorporate the KidScents products on page 51. If you want to take it up a notch, you may want to incorporate the Raindrop products. (See page 44.)

(Give the guests a few minutes to develop their plan. Be available to help them personalize, otherwise, sit back, be quiet and let them think.)

Okay, now that you all have your plan, pull out your smartphone and log onto your Shopping Platform. We are going to set up your first month's order with Subscribe to Save. If you are not familiar with this yet, this will save you money while getting the products you need to get well. Remember, if you order more than 50pv you will earn free products through our Loyalty Rewards program too. All you have to do is make sure you consistently process 50pv every month to participate. I have your member number if you don't know it.

(Coach them through setting up their order. You can send the guests a link to the My YL Bundle that corresponds with their health goal. Help them navigate the shopping platform and create their account.)

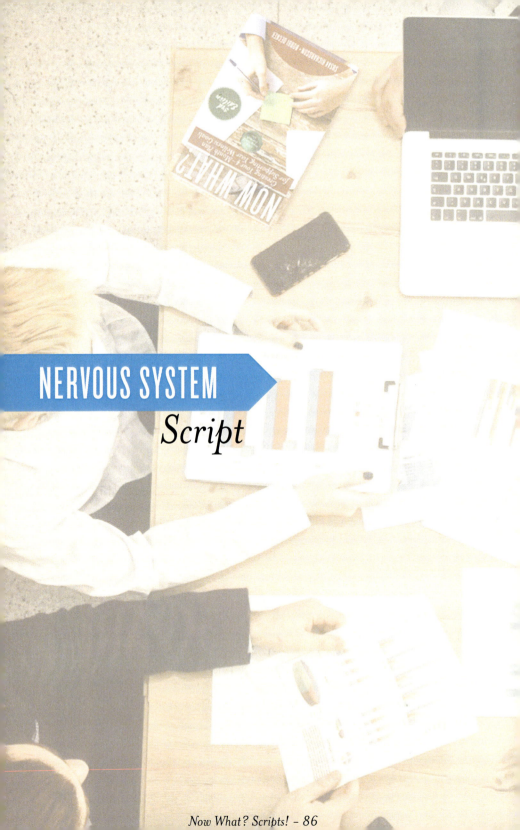

NERVOUS SYSTEM
Script

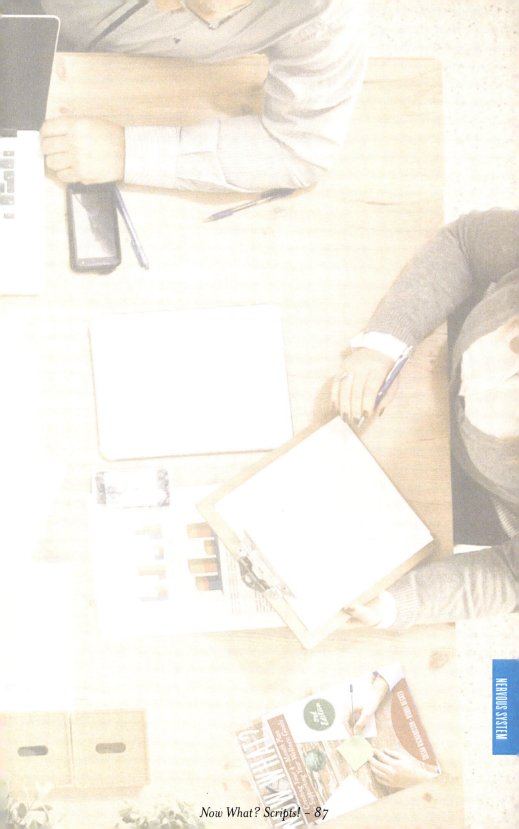

NERVOUS SYSTEM

Hello everyone, in case you don't know me, my name is _____ . I am part of your Young Living Support Team. Thank you for being a part of our oily family. I want to thank (Host/Hostess) for opening up his/her home to us so we can learn more about how to take your health to the next level.

As Young Living customers, we all know what essential oils are and how they work in our bodies. Essential oils and essential oil-infused products are the number one way to protect your home from harsh chemicals and toxins; and promote health for you and your entire family.

Because Young Living is a health and wellness company, we are able to address wellness from a whole body perspective. And we can also look more in-depth at individual body systems like we are going to do today with the nervous system.

This shouldn't shock you, but we discourage people from buying just a single oil. However, if that is what you choose, we recommend you put it on a Subscribe to Save oder to help you save money. We don't want to mislead anyone into thinking one bottle of oil can help them achieve their health goals. Instead, we like to empower you with healthy lifestyle habits and to set up your own 4-Month Wellness Plan so you can reach and maintain your health goals.

With all of this in mind, let's take a close look at the nervous system and discuss a few ways to address this system of the body so you can keep it above the health line.

So, open your Now What? book to the Nervous System on page 22. This system collects and processes information from the nerves in the brain. The autonomic nervous system controls involuntary activities such as heartbeat, breathing, digestion, glandular activities and the blood vessels. This system is greatly affected by the digestive system.

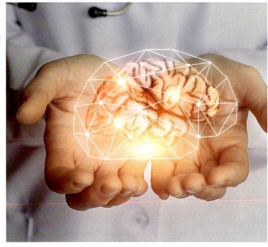

Do you have a mediocre diet? (Wait for a yes.)

Have you ever been so busy that you forgot to eat a meal? (Wait for a yes.)

This isn't good for your body or your brain. It is SO important to do everything you can to ensure you and your family are getting the proper nutrition you need to support every system of your body.

We know that when we use an essential oil-infused product, it helps our body absorb and distribute nutrition from the foods we eat and makes the nutrients from our supplements we take more bioavailable. We can even use the Vitality essential oils as dietary supplements. You should already have some Vitality oils and Classic Essential Oils. Whatever you have, make sure you pull them out and use them every day. We recommend you get Frankincense, Lavender and Lemon Vitality, if you don't already have them.

You can easily add a drop of Lavender and Frankincense Vitality to your morning NingXia Red shot to support your nervous system.

So let's all do a NingXia shot while we discuss NingXia Red. (Pass nervous system shots around.)

NingXia Red supports every system of the body, even for those of us who are already healthy. NingXia Red helps us to maintain that health, stamina, and cognitive wellness.

It is a funny name, but NingXia is actually the name of the province in China where the primary ingredient is grown. The NingXia wolfberry is the predominant food of the people in this region who live to be over 100 years old. They contribute their health and longevity to this particular wolfberry which is packed full of dense nutrition and contains 4x the nutrients of the wolfberries in neighboring provinces.

NingXia Red is very high in antioxidants, which means that it helps support our body's natural defense against aging. Dr. Richard Cutler of the National Institutes of Health said, "The amount of antioxidants that you maintain in your body is directly proportional to how long you live!" Consuming antioxidants is an excellent way to slow down the effects of aging on the brain and to improve cognitive skills.

There are actually 17 species of wolfberry and only the NingXia wolfberry has a complete phytonutrient profile. It is higher in vitamin C than oranges, higher in beta-carotene than carrots, and higher in calcium than cauliflower. Calcium is necessary for healthy brain function and for the neurotransmitters to fire correctly.

NingXia Red is also high in vitamin E and protein. It is a good source of amino acids and 21 trace minerals which are important for all of the body systems to properly function. It also has 6 essential fatty acids which is important because our body cannot make essential fatty acids; they must come from our diet.

NingXia Red also has vitamins B1, B2, & B6 and more. This is dense nutrition. And let's face it, most people are not getting what they need from the food they eat.

It contains high quality juices and purees like blueberry, pomegranate, plum, and cherry. Amazingly, even with these juices included, it still supports healthy blood sugar levels and offers low glycemic energy. This is because it is a puree and contains the fruit fiber. NingXia Red contains a patented grape seed extract that contains polyphenolic compounds that may help support a healthy cardiovascular system as well.

Another thing that sets NingXia Red apart is that it is the only nutritive supplement available that is infused with essential oils. This aids the body's ability to absorb and assimilate all of those nutrients offering whole body support including our emotional well-being.

Let's talk a little bit about physical activity because while diet and nutrition are important, it's good to move your body. The American Heart Association recommends for a healthy heart you need to get 150 minutes of moderate exercise a week. Being physically active is important in preventing heart disease and stroke. Just 30 minutes of walking a day will decrease your chances of falling below the health line. So let's all stand up and move. Change seats and sit by someone new. Seriously, let's get up and move.

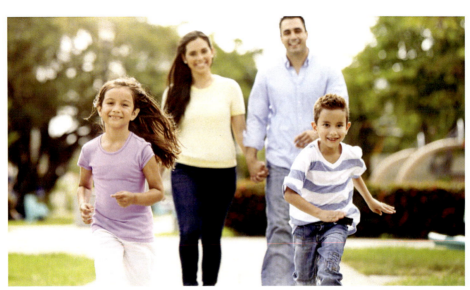

4-MONTH WELLNESS PLAN

NingXia Red is the foundation for every system of the body, so it stands to reason that it is the first addition to your 4-Month Wellness Plan. It doesn't matter what your goal is, this is our #1 choice for everyone.

Let's also talk about MindWise. This is an AMAZING supplement that everyone should be taking along with their NingXia Red. MindWise proprietary memory blend features ALCAR. According to the National Library of Medicine, Acetyl-l-carnitine (ALCAR), is a substance which has been shown to prevent some impairments of the aged central nervous system or CNS. Supplementation with ALCAR completely prevents the loss of choline activity in the CNS.

MindWise also has GPC (alpha glycerylphosphorylcholine), a natural physiological precursor to a neurotransmitter that is one of the best known cognitive enhancers. This neurotransmitter is involved in memory and other cognitive functions and is known to cross the blood brain barrier. Clinical studies have demonstrated it helps to support cognitive function and mental acuity. It is a form of choline which plays an important role in cell signaling and neurotransmission. There is scientific consensus that choline reserves in the human body are depleted as we age, leading to a decreased neurological activity in most adults.

MindWise also has CoQ10 which is found in every cell of the body and is necessary for the basic functioning of cells and has been studied for supporting healthy brain function.

MindWise contains medium chain triglycerides (MCT) from coconut oil and generous amounts of vitamin D3. MCT is readily known in scientific communities as "Rocket Fuel for the Brain." MCTs are essential for the development of babies' brains and are found in abundance in human breast milk. MCT oil provides an easily absorbed source of energy for those with food absorption difficulties. MCTs are unique among fats since they don't require bile salts for digestion or extra energy for absorption, use, or storage. Everybody benefits from this.

To complement NingXia Red and MindWise, we have a supplement called Mineral Essence which is a balanced full spectrum ionic mineral complex enhanced with essential oils. According to two-time Nobel Prize winner Linus Pauling Ph.D., "You can trace every sickness, every disease, and every ailment to a mineral deficiency." Ionic minerals are the most fully and quickly absorbed form of minerals available.

Mineral Essence contains honey; honey has been praised as the optimum fuel for the brain. It is known to prevent metabolic stress and help with restful sleep. This in turn is critical for our cognitive and memory enhancement. And, YES, ancient people held the belief that honey had the ability to boost memory, intellect, and concentration. Little did they know how right they were. There is now a body of scientific evidence to support their beliefs.

The minerals contained in royal jelly are iron, calcium, copper, potassium, phosphorus, silicon, and sulfur. Another compound delivered is acetylcholine (which we have mentioned a few times today). This neurotransmitter is directly related to the quality of memory, thought, concentration, and focus. It almost acts as a sort of lubricant at the nerve cell junctions and is a part of the nervous system.

Another supplement and great complimentary product also combining Vitamin D3, CoQ10 and fatty acids is OmegaGize3. This supplement is infused with DHA-rich fish oil and essential oils which work synergistically to support normal brain function.

Need a quick cognitive boost without a crash? Next time grab your NingXia Nitro! This supplement is infused with essential oils, botanical extracts, D-ribose, Korean ginseng, and green tea extract. This product supports alertness, as well as cognitive and physical fitness.

As we all know, stress is a familiar part of daily life, but did you know AMINO ACIDS support your brain chemistry and promote positive emotions when dealing with anxiety, fear, worry, panic and feelings of stress or just being overwhelmed with life?

WHO KNEW!!!! Drink up your AminoWise today!!!!

"When you balance your brain chemistry, not only will you alleviate symptoms of anxiety, you'll also have a great mood, eliminate cravings, sleep well, and have good energy and mental focus," Food Mood Expert, Trudy Scott, Nutritionist

A complementary essential oil blend for the nervous system is Brain Power. Brain Power is formulated with essential oils that are high in sesquiterpenes to promote clarity and focus when diffused or applied. You can apply this on your temples, across your forehead or even on the back of your neck to enhance your mental acuity.

We also recommend the Thieves clean living line. This line includes the Thieves essential oil blend and products infused with this blend including the household cleaner, hand soap, toothpaste, mouthwash, hand sanitizer and even a misting spray to conveniently use when you are out and about. These products are going to replace all of your cleaning supplies and many of your personal care items that impede your brain function and nervous system.

It is super easy to integrate them into your daily lifestyle by ordering them through Young Living's Subscribe to Save program. Just select the products you want, the frequency you want them, and have them shipped to your front door.

This product line is safe enough to use around our children and pets. We can use this household cleaner on everything from lunch boxes to toilets. This plant based formula uses a naturally occurring surfactant derived from coconut and is non abrasive, leaves behind no chemical residue and is safe for septic systems. It is highly concentrated, making it cost effective! (Hold up pre-diluted spray bottle.) This bottle is my all purpose cleaner. I add one cap of the Thieves Household Cleaner and fill the rest with water. I use this on everything.

By using these products, you will protect your home from harsh chemicals that can compromise your health while saving you money. And, it doesn't matter if you are brushing your teeth or scrubbing your toilet, you are supporting your health when you use any of the Thieves products.

The NON-Young Living personal care products that we are buying in box stores such as laundry detergent, lotions, shampoos, bath and body products and even oils are made with harsh chemicals and fragrances. These are made in factories and laboratories, not grown in a field. The toxins from these other products compromise not only our nervous system, but every system of the body.

In the same way, every time we wash our dishes, we are absorbing chemicals like sodium lauryl sulfate which can be in a ratio as high as 30%. This level is considered unsafe and is affecting us. This is not just in your dish soap but is also found in toothpaste, mouthwash, makeup, body wash and shampoos. Sodium lauryl sulfate *(SLS) is known to be a "moderate hazard" and has been linked to cancer, neurotoxicity, organ toxicity, skin irritation and endocrine disruption; and yet it is one of the most commonly used ingredients in shampoos.*

Young Living has many safe products to increase your ability to nourish your hair and skin. Remember when you are in a hot shower, your pores open up, so what you are shampooing with will absorb into your body when it runs down your body. You can rest assured that all of Young Living's shampoos and conditioners are plant derived and safe and formulated to leave your hair healthy and clean. There also may be an adjustment time with the personal care products as we switch from harsh products to plant-based ingredients. Young Living products are super concentrated, so less is more.

The products we covered today are great examples of what you can put on your Subscribe to Save order to jump start your 4-Month Wellness Plan. But remember, everybody is different, sometimes we have an immediate response using Young Living products, but I am sure we all can agree that one drop of oil will not really support the underlying signals your body may be giving you. You need to make a commitment to use your products consistently. Be okay with that.

You've already started by being here. Now use your NOW WHAT? book to set up a 4-Month Wellness Plan. Write down your own personalized plan on the "My Order" spaces on page 23.

And remember to personalize your choices. Look at the Complementary Products and choose from there too. If you are personalizing for a child, you may want to incorporate the Kidscents products on page 43. If you want to take it up a notch, you may want to incorporate the Neuro Auricular Technique or NAT.

(Give the guests a few minutes to develop their plan. Be available to help them personalize, otherwise, sit back, be quiet and let them think.)

Okay, now that you all have your plan, pull out your smartphone and log onto your Shopping Platform. We are going to set up your first Subscribe to Save order.
If you are not familiar with this yet, this will save you money while getting the products you need to get well. Remember, if you order more than 50pv you will earn free products through our Loyalty Rewards program too. All you have to do is make sure you consistently process 50pv every month to participate. I have your member number if you don't know it.

(Coach them through setting up their order. You can send the guests a link to the My YL Bundle that corresponds with their health goal. Help them navigate the shopping platform and create their account.)

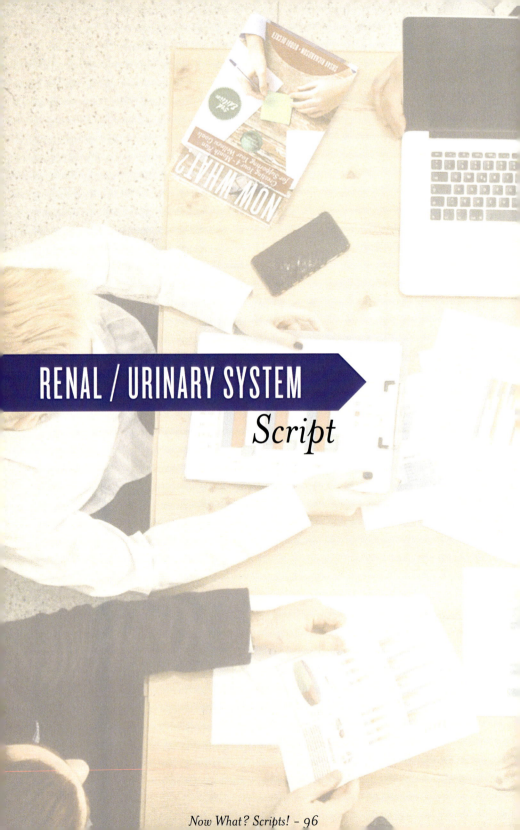

RENAL / URINARY SYSTEM
Script

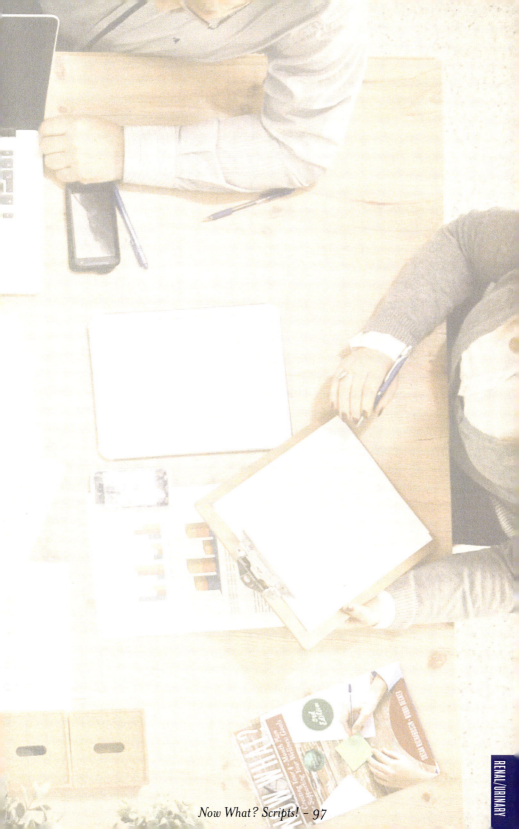

RENAL / URINARY SYSTEM

Hello everyone, in case you don't know me, my name is _____ . I am part of your Young Living Support Team. Thank you for being a part of our oily family. I want to thank (Host/Hostess) for opening up his/her home to us so we can learn more about how to take your health to the next level.

As Young Living customers, we all know what essential oils are and how they work in our bodies. Essential oils and essential oil-infused products are the number one way to protect your home from harsh chemicals and toxins; and promote health for you and your entire family.

Because Young Living is a health and wellness company, we are able to address wellness from a whole body perspective. And we can also look more in-depth at individual body systems, like we are going to do today with the urinary system.

This shouldn't shock you, but we discourage people from buying just a single oil. However, if that is what you choose, we recommend you put it on a Subscribe to Save oder to help you save money. We don't want to mislead anyone into thinking one bottle of oil can help them achieve their health goals. Instead, we like to empower you with healthy lifestyle habits and to set up your own 4-Month Wellness Plan so you can reach and maintain your health goals.

With all this in mind, let's take a closer look at the urinary system and discuss a few ways to address this system of the body so you can keep it above the health line. With all this in mind, let's take a closer look at the urinary system and discuss a few ways to address this system of the body so you can keep it above the health line.

So, open your Now What? book to the Renal/ Urinary System on page 24 and 25. This system is where the kidneys filter the blood and remove waste products and maintain normalized blood pressure. When you stay above the health line, your kidneys filter 200 quarts of blood every day and remove more than 2 quarts of waste that flow through the bladder.

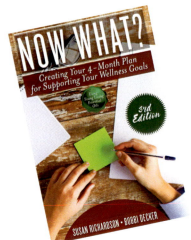

It is SO important to do everything you can to ensure you and your family are getting the proper nutrition you need to support this system of the body and every other system, too.

We know that when we use an essential oil-infused product it helps our bodies absorb and distribute nutrition from the foods we eat and makes the nutrients from our supplements we take more bioavailable. We can even use the Vitality essential oils as dietary supplements. You should already have some Vitality oils and Classic Essential Oils. Whatever you have, make sure you pull them out and use them every day. We recommend you get Lemon, Grapefruit and Frankincense Vitality, if you don't already have them. Lemon and Grapefruit Vitality are perfect additions to your water and help keep your body's pH levels in balance. You can easily add a drop of each to your morning NingXia Red shot to support your urinary system. So let's all

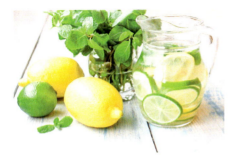

do a NingXia shot while we discuss NingXia Red. *(Pass urinary shots around.)*
NingXia Red supports every system of the body. Even for those of us who are already healthy. NingXia Red helps us to maintain that health, stamina, and cognitive wellness.

It is a funny name, but Ningxia is actually the name of the province in China where the primary ingredient is grown. The Ningxia wolfberry is the predominant food of the people in this region who live to be over 100 years old. They contribute their health and longevity to this particular wolfberry which is packed full of dense nutrition and contains 4x the nutrients of the wolfberries in neighboring provinces.

NingXia Red is very high in antioxidants, which means that it helps support our body's natural defense against aging. Dr. Richard Cutler of the National Institutes of Health said, "The amount of antioxidants that you maintain in your body is directly proportional to how long you live!" In addition, oxidative stress plays a role in disease and infections. So it stands to reason that we want to be sure we have adequate antioxidants in our diet.

There are actually 17 species of wolfberry but only the Ningxia wolfberry has a complete phytonutrient profile. It is higher in vitamin C than oranges, higher in beta-carotene than carrots and higher in calcium than cauliflower. Calcium is responsible for functions in the body like regulating normal blood pressure. And there is ample research on the health benefits of vitamin C and the urinary tract. The vitamin C turns the urine acidic and creates an unfriendly terrain for bacteria.

NingXia Red is also high in vitamin E and protein. The wolfberries are a good source of amino acids and 21 trace minerals which are important for all of the systems of the body to properly function. It also has 6 essential fatty acids which is important because our body cannot make essential fatty acids, they must come from our diet.

NingXia Red also has vitamins B1, B2, and B6. The body utilizes B vitamins to produce red blood cells, hormone production and more. If you want an extra vitamin B boost, look at Super B™. This is a comprehensive B complex containing ALL 8 B vitamins including folate that is sourced from lemon peels to make it more bioavailable. These Bs are in the best possible ratio to be absorbed by your body and contain folate which is vital for normal kidney and bladder function.

This is dense nutrition. And let's face it, most people are not getting what they need from the food they eat.

NingXia Red also contains high quality juices and purees like blueberry, pomegranate, plum, and cherry. Amazingly, even with these juices included, it still supports healthy blood sugar levels and offers low glycemic energy. This is because it is a puree and contains the fruit fiber.

NingXia Red contains a patented grape seed extract that contains polyphenolic compounds that have been studied for renal health.

Another thing that sets NingXia Red apart is that it is the only nutritive supplement available that is infused with essential oils. This aids the body's ability to absorb and assimilate all of those nutrients offering whole body support including our emotional well-being.
We have discussed NingXia Red and that it is the foundation for every system so it stands to reason that it is the first addition to your 4-Month Wellness Plan. It doesn't matter what your goal is, this is our #1 choice for everyone.

Let's talk a little bit about physical activity because while diet and nutrition are important, it's good to move your body. The American Kidney Foundation recommends 30 minutes of moderate exercise a day. Being physically active is important in preventing kidney disease and improves overall wellness. Just 30 minutes of walking a day will decrease your chances of falling below the health line. So let's all stand up and move. Change seats and sit by someone new. Seriously, let's get up and move.

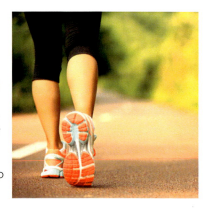

4-MONTH WELLNESS PLAN

K & B is a tincture specifically formulated to maintain kidney & bladder health and enhance the body's efforts to maintain fluid balance. It is infused with the extracts of juniper, parsley, and dandelion root, all of which are thought to be natural cleansers and purifiers. K & B also has Uva Ursi Leaf extract which is known to maintain the pH balance of urine. When the pH is alkaline, it keeps the natural inflammatory response at bay. This tincture combines these herbs with royal jelly and pure essential oils to not only support a healthy renal system, but to strengthen it as well.

As we know, all health begins in the digestive system. And the health of your circulatory system and renal system is directly linked to the health of your gut in that they work together to create homeostasis in your body. So, along with NingXia Red and K&B, Life 9 is a great supplement to use. Life 9 is pretty amazing because it has 9 clinically proven high-potency probiotic strains that work well together. It combines 17 billion live cultures from these 9 bacteria strains that promote healthy digestion, support gut health and help maintain normal intestinal function for overall health.

Balance Complete is a powerful nutritive cleanser that contains a V-fiber blend that absorbs toxins and contains folate for renal system protection.

Inner Defense and ImmuPro are perfect companions for your renal 4-Month Wellness Plan. Inner Defense enhances your immune system and renal system. It is basically Thieves Vitality in a capsule combined with the proper ratio of Thyme Vitality, Oregano Vitality and Lemongrass Vitality for extra support. Inner Defense creates an unfriendly terrain for yeast and fungus in your gut. It tends to be most effective when taken 6-8 hours before our probiotic, Life 9.

ImmuPro is a chewable that also gives unprecedented immune support, but also promotes restful sleep. Your physical and mental health can be directly affected by the quality of your sleep patterns. ImmuPro reinforces this.

The products we covered today are great examples of what you can put on your Subscribe to Save order to jump start your 4-Month Wellness Plan. But remember, everybody is different, sometimes we have an immediate response using Young Living products, but I am sure we all can agree that one drop of oil will not really support the underlying signals your body may be giving you. You need to make a commitment to use your products consistently. Be okay with that.

You've already started by being here. Now use your NOW WHAT? book to set up a 4-Month Wellness Plan. Check off the products you want to order each month on page 25.

And remember to personalize your choices. Look at the "You May Also Like" Products and choose from there, too.

(Give the guests a few minutes to develop their plan. Be available to help them personalize, otherwise, sit back, be quiet and let them think.)

Okay, now that you all have your plan, pull out your smartphone and log into your Shopping Platform. We are going to set up your first month's order with Subscribe to Save. This will save you money while getting the products you need to get well. Remember, if you order more than 50pv you will earn free products through our Loyalty Rewards program too. All you have to do is make sure you consistently process 50pv every month to participate. I have your member number if you don't know it.

(Coach them through setting up their order. You can send the guests a link to the My YL Bundle that corresponds with their health goal. Help them navigate the shopping platform and create their account.)

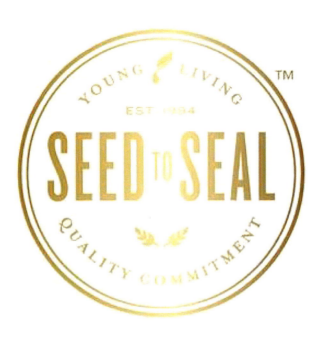